O^{THE}rgasm LOOP

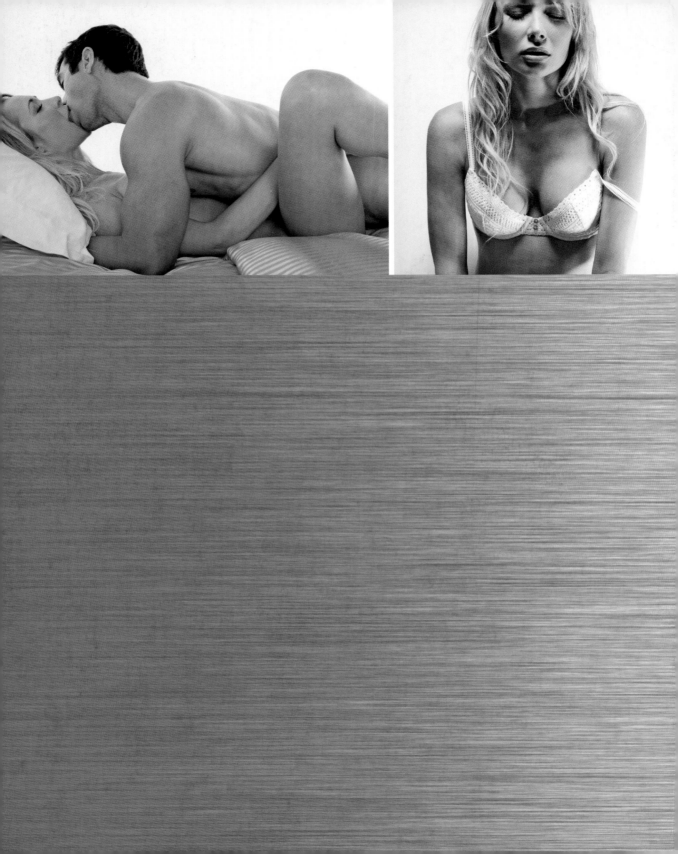

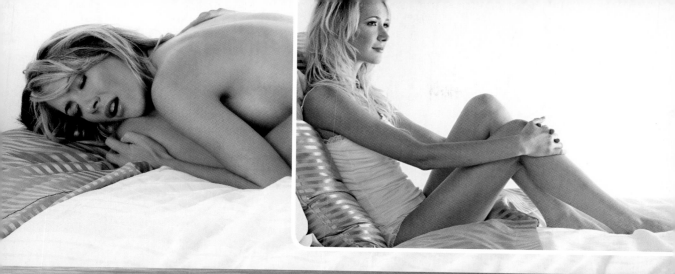

THE Orgasm LOOP

The No-Fail Technique
for Reaching Orgasm During Sex

Susan Crain Bakos

QUIVER

Text © 2008 Susan Crain Bakos
Photography © 2008 Quiver

First published in the USA in 2008 by
Quiver, a member of
Quayside Publishing Group
100 Cummings Center
Suite 406-L
Beverly, MA 01915-6101
www.quiverbooks.com

The Publisher maintains the records relating to images in this book required
by 18 USC 2257. Records are located at Rockport Publishers, Inc.,
100 Cummings Center, Suite 406-L, Beverly, MA 01915-6101.

12 11 10 09 08   1 2 3 4 5

ISBN-13: 978-1-59233-333-2
ISBN-10: 1-59233-333-8

Library of Congress Cataloging-in-Publication Data available
Bakos, Susan Crain.
The orgasm loop : the no-fail technique for reaching orgasm during sex / Susan Crain Bakos.
    p. cm.
ISBN 1-59233-333-8
1. Sex instruction. 2. Orgasm. I. Title.
HQ31.B234964 2008
613.9'6082--dc22
                           2007044059

Cover and book design: Holtz Design

Printed and bound in Singapore

DEDICATION
This book is for my late sister, Ellen, who was always a little embarrassed about the sex thing but proud of me anyway. She gave me my wings.

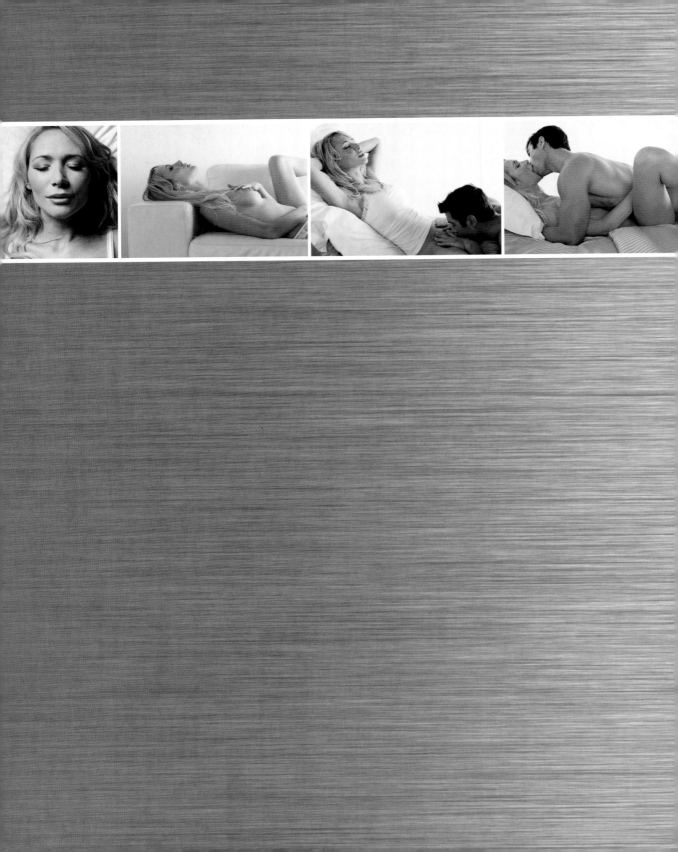

Contents

Introduction

For every woman, there is an orgasm.

Yet it often remains elusive. Millions of women have difficulty reaching orgasm. That was true before the Sexual Revolution, the Women's Revolution, women-friendly porn, and sex toy parties in the suburbs—and it's true now. And, yes, women are still faking the orgasms they aren't having. Are you living your grandmother's sex life?

Not all women are in this same orgasm place. Some have little or no difficulty reaching orgasm with their partners. Others reach orgasm easily through masturbation but not so easily during lovemaking. Still others come via cunnilingus or manual stimulation, but can't get there during intercourse alone.

What are the REAL Numbers on Women and Orgasm?

- Approximately 65 percent of women need additional clitoral stimulation during intercourse to reach orgasm that way.
- And 10 to 20 percent of women seldom or never reach orgasm.

The "seldom or never" group added to the "I don't want to touch myself during sex" faction of the "no orgasm during intercourse" group creates that large pool of "dissatisfied women" cited by research studies and survey polls. Remember the often-quoted 1999 study in *The Journal of the American Medical Association* that claimed 43 percent of women were sexually dissatisfied? However the data is sliced, a significant number of women wish their sex lives were better—or, worse, don't believe they ever will have the kind of pleasure they read about and see in films. Why is orgasm a "maybe" for a significant portion of women?

One, Two, Three—and You're Not There

Here's how the Female Orgasm Strike-Out works:

First, intercourse is designed for male orgasm, the biological imperative for reproduction. (Her biological imperative? Lie there.) He comes through the friction of his penis moving inside her vagina. Intercourse alone doesn't work for most women because they need direct clitoral stimulation to reach orgasm—and the clitoris is outside the vagina.

Secondly, many women are uncomfortable touching themselves during sex. As little girls, they were told not to touch themselves "down there." (Boys get the same message, but they discard it more easily for the obvious reason: the penis is outside the body tempting them.)

Often, many women don't want to touch themselves during sex because they feel it takes away from the romance and makes sex too mechanical, as if they're just doing what it takes to get the job done, instead of allowing passion, love, and emotional connection with their partner to get the job done for them. A woman wants to think her Prince's magic wand is sufficient, and she wants her Prince to think the same.

The third strike? The myth that intimacy trumps orgasms. According to this misconception, women would rather feel close and connected to their partners than come. A study reported in a CNN story in November 2006 was one of many claiming it's not orgasm, but intimacy, that women crave. Decades of female sexual empowerment have been casually swept aside by the reiteration of that old lie. Yes, women want to feel close and connected to their partners—but they, just like men, feel closer and more strongly connected after orgasm. It's the endorphin high. Orgasm releases a flood of feel-good chemicals that elevates your mood and makes you feel more bonded to your partner.

The Orgasm Bottom Line

How can I have an orgasm during intercourse?

This is women's number-one sex concern, the question they constantly ask of magazine and online columnists, sex therapists, and educators. It was the number-one sex question to *Cosmopolitan* magazine under the legendary Helen Gurley Brown for decades. And Kate White, current editor-in-chief of *Cosmopolitan* magazine, says it is still the number-one sex question the magazine gets from readers. On a daily basis, I see research studies and reader surveys about female sexual behavior that follow women from age eighteen to fifty, and the topic is too often FSD, female sexual dysfunction: women reporting low desire and difficulties reaching orgasm. The problem is not that women are "dysfunctional." Women are *disappointed* in sex because they believe that intercourse alone should lead to orgasm for them the same way it does for men. And then they blame themselves and/or their partners when it doesn't happen.

The prevalence of The Question and the overwhelming evidence that low or no desire is the biggest sex issue for women in relationships are facts that can't be reconciled with the myth of women preferring intimacy over orgasms. When women say they don't care whether they come or not, frankly, I don't believe them. They mean: I *probably won't come so I'm not interested in sex*. If intimacy were truly their number-one desire, wouldn't they always say "yes" to sex to get close?

That's why I began looking for a revolutionary technique that could give any woman an orgasm any time she wants one. I expected to find it somewhere in books on Tantric sex, the Eastern lovemaking arts defined by the Kama Sutra. But nothing I discovered in those books or others, in research studies, or during interviews with easily orgasmic women gave me the answer.

So I invented the Orgasm Loop, a revolutionary mind-body technique for removing the mental roadblocks to orgasm. The Orgasm Loop taps into a woman's arousal potential and teaches her how to use her body to her own best orgasm advantage.

I've tested the Loop on 575 women to date—with overwhelmingly positive results. In the summer of 2007, noted neuroscientist Dr. Barry Komisaruk and famous sexologist Dr. Beverly Whipple, authors of *The Science of Orgasm*, tested the Orgasm Loop technique in research conducted through the University of Medicine and Dentistry of Rutgers University (New Jersey, U.S.). Women testing the Loop did reach orgasm, lighting up the orgasm areas of their brains on fMRI scans (magnetic resonance imagery, or brain scans). It was the first time Kegel exercises were used by women in fMRI-based studies.

The first few times you use the Orgasm Loop, you'll have to think about what you're doing. You will need to focus more on achieving arousal and getting your own pleasure than on your partner. (He won't mind. The results will be worth it for both of you, because a man's number-one desire is to "give" his partner an orgasm.) After that, the technique comes naturally—as will your orgasms during intercourse, masturbation, or other kinds of sex play. This book will guide you through the stages of learning the Orgasm Loop and adding it to every phase of your sex life, so you can always focus on your arousal and reach orgasm every time.

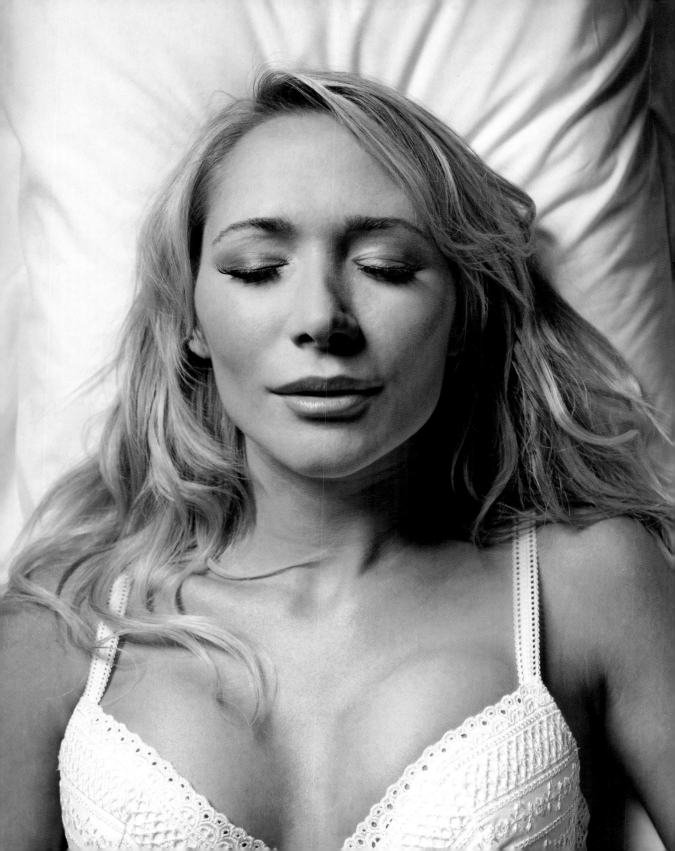

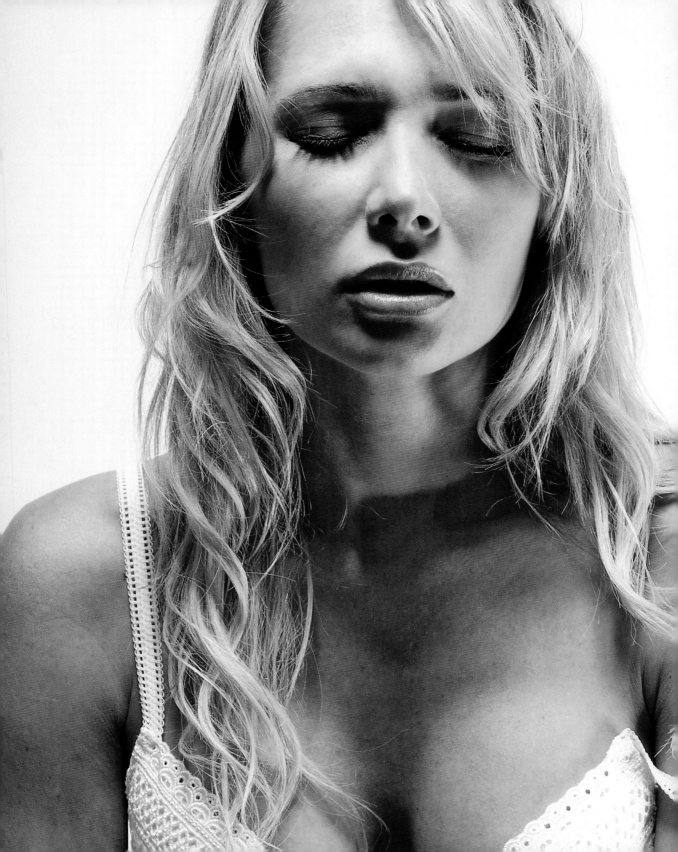

Part 1

The Orgasm Loop

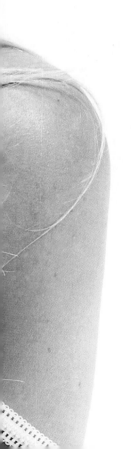

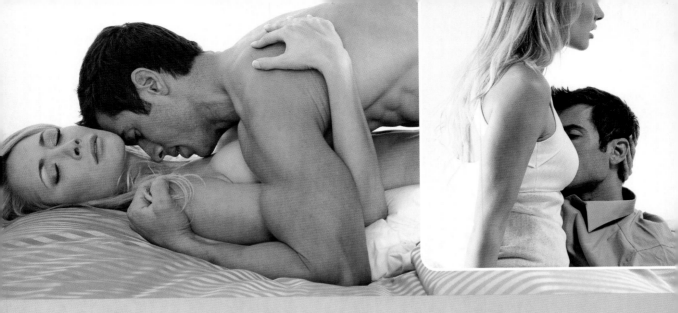

Chapter 1
The New Theory of Orgasm

"The !Kung bushmen [of the Kalahari Desert in Africa] believe that a woman who does not have regular sex and orgasms will lose her mind and end up eating grass and dying."

—Dr. Jonathan Margolis, author of
O: The Intimate History of the Orgasm

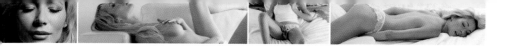

WHY IS ORGASM SO IMPORTANT? Why not accept the ubiquitous, "Really, it's just closeness I crave" excuse? Why not give up on women who just won't touch themselves during intercourse?

Orgasm is the most intense physical pleasure we ever have. Nothing else comes close. Incredibly, the average orgasmic person, male or female, only spends approximately twelve minutes a year in the throes of orgasm. Really, that is not enough. Yet women accept even less. No wonder we buy so many pairs of shoes!

Given the power and glory that is orgasm, I've never accepted the status quo thinking that holds that his orgasm is inevitable while hers is problematic. Why should female orgasm be problematic when we are the possessors of the clitoris, which is richer with more concentrated nerve endings than any part of his body? Why should female orgasm be problematic when we are capable of multiple orgasms with no refractory period? And besides, we are the gender who really gets better (in terms of sexual response), not older.

Every woman should have an orgasm—at least one!—every day of her life.

A Brief History of the Quest for the Big O

The list of theories on female orgasm that were once fashionable usually begins with Freud, who said, "The clitoral orgasm is immature, the vaginal orgasm, mature"—thus setting the impossible standard for modern women. Up until the second half of the twentieth century, it was deemed even more desirable under certain circumstances, like being married, for women to reach orgasm—but still in the ideal way via "unassisted" intercourse (in other words, intercourse with no additional clitoral stimulation—a sort of sexual Holy Grail).

Research conducted in the 1960s by Dr. William Masters and Dr. Virginia Johnson on male and female sexuality changed the status quo. In their books, beginning with *Human Sexual Response* in 1966, they asserted that most women reach orgasm via clitoral stimulation. Suddenly, "clitoro-centrism" ruled. Then, in the 1980s, Dr. Beverly Whipple and her

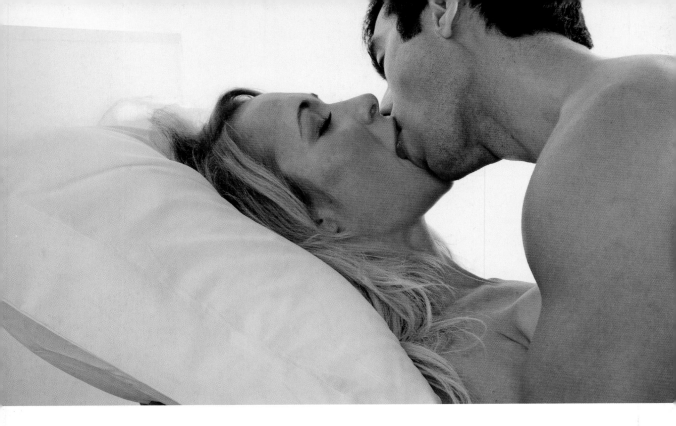

cohorts introduced the G-spot orgasm, a salvo in defense of the vaginal orgasm. And Dr. Ian Kerner countered with the doctrine of "clitoracy" in his 2004 tutorial on cunnilingus, *She Comes First.*

The clitoris—out, in, out, in again.

Yet, regardless of these changing trends, the question for women has remained the same: How can I come during intercourse?

"We found that some women really noticed when their genitals were aroused and these women were orgasmic—while others barely paid attention to genital swelling or lubricating and generally were not orgasmic."

—Dr. Julia Heiman, psychology professor and director of the Kinsey Institute, regarding the Pfizer female Viagra studies she conducted

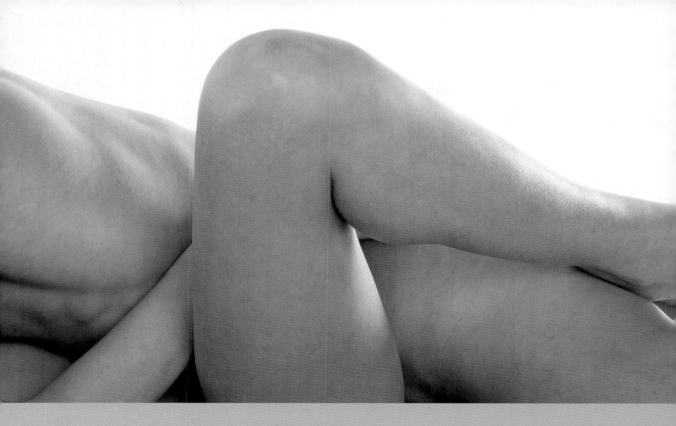

Real Talk

THE QUEST FOR THE HOLY O

"I can orgasm during lovemaking—if he uses his hand or his
tongue. We have these you-first-now-me orgasms. Have
I ever come during intercourse alone? No. And that is
the Holy Grail to me. I want to come with him inside me, I want
to come when he comes, I want to really feel it, not just fake it
occasionally."

—Jessica, 28

The New Theory of Orgasm: "It's All in Your Head."

Recent studies have concluded that most of women's difficulties with arousal (and thus orgasm) are mental. Women have difficulty recognizing their own physical arousal and connecting the subtle signs of arousal in their minds with the desire for sex. A study conducted at Tulane University in New Orleans measured arousal by accelerated heart rate and breathing, erection in men, and vasocongestion (swelling of the genitals) and lubrication in women. The authors of the study reported that women are aroused as easily and as often as men by erotic imagery—*but they ignore their arousal.* According to another study conducted at Washington University in St. Louis based on fMRI scans, sexy images actually enter the female's brain faster than they do the male's brain. Yet men report arousal in these controlled environments far more often than women do. These results became international news when they were released in early 2007.

What's happening in women's brains to short-circuit arousal? Sometimes, the part of the brain that delivers negative sexual messages—from "that's too naughty" to "you're too fat for that"—overrides the arousal. Often women simply ignore their genitals and whatever they are trying to tell them. We women are our own worst sexual enemies. We worry too much about the wrong things, like how we compare to supermodels' bodies, instead of focusing on the sex itself. Many women don't really focus on orgasm until they are having intercourse—and then they believe that it doesn't happen because they are "trying too hard."

The Arousal Disparity

Arousal works in different ways for men and women, and the signs are a lot more obvious to men. "A man receives cognitive feedback from his erection," says Dr. Eileen Palace, director of the Center for Sexual Health in New Orleans. "Women … have tingling, throbbing, and lubrication, but it's very subtle, and you can't see it. To fully enjoy sex a woman needs something that links what's happening down below to the brain."

A man gets an erection and he knows he wants to have sex because the male erection/brain connection, aided by the visual element, is strong. Dr. Eileen Palace calls this mind-body connection the Cognitive Physiological Feedback Loop (CPFL). A woman's genitals don't always get the arousal message to her brain, in part because the signs of female arousal are more subtle. Often she has sex without fully tapping into her arousal, thus making orgasm problematic.

In addition, any number of common mental roadblocks get in her way and put a damper on arousal. She allows herself to become distracted by body issues, performance concerns, relationship issues, stress, tension, and worry—and loses her arousal, at least for a time, again making orgasm problematic.

Men don't seem to hit these sorts of roadblocks where sex is concerned. They are naturally erotically self-involved. And that's NOT a bad thing! They get past the self—what the penis wants—to make the emotional connection with a woman when sex is working for them. If women could put erotic self-involvement ahead of the concepts of "relationship," "love," "intimacy," and "Do my breasts sag in this position?" then we too would get the pleasure *and* make the emotional connection that often gets lost because the sex isn't working for us.

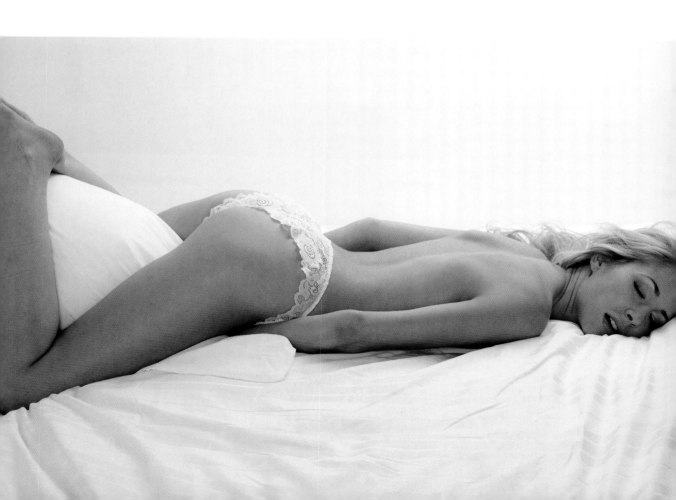

Entering the Loop

Influenced by the cognitive feedback loop studies conducted by Dr. Palace, I began to research techniques for removing the mental roadblocks to arousal. I wanted to take her arousal studies a step further by showing women how to recognize, visualize, and encourage their suppressed arousal. In the fMRI studies at Rutgers University, women see their arousal on screens. The scans show the blood flow to the brain during arousal and orgasm as lighted areas.

Women who think they are not aroused can see their own arousal—and when they see it, they start to feel it. It was suddenly so clear to me: *men see their arousal. Women don't see theirs. Thus, we need to visualize it.* I watched these fMRI scans in progress and also witnessed biofeedback arousal studies where women were connected to devices that monitor heart rate, genital swelling, and lubrication with the same, though less visually spectacular, results. And I knew I could take women to this place of visualizing arousal without machines.

To enjoy sex fully, a woman needs something that links what's happening down below to the brain—a visual image that can become as potent as the sight of his erection is to him. That became step one of the Orgasm Loop: a woman needs to create a unique arousal image in her mind and use it every time. An arousal image of an open flower, like an orchid, has been effective for some women. (You'll learn more on how a woman creates this arousal image when you read Chapter 2, "How the O Loop Works.")

"I had my first orgasm at 30. When that first orgasm happened, it wasn't some skilled lover boy who showed me how; it was me."

—Hilda Hutcherson, M.D., author of *Pleasure: A Woman's Guide to Getting the Sex You Want, Need and Deserve* and advice columnist for *Glamour* magazine

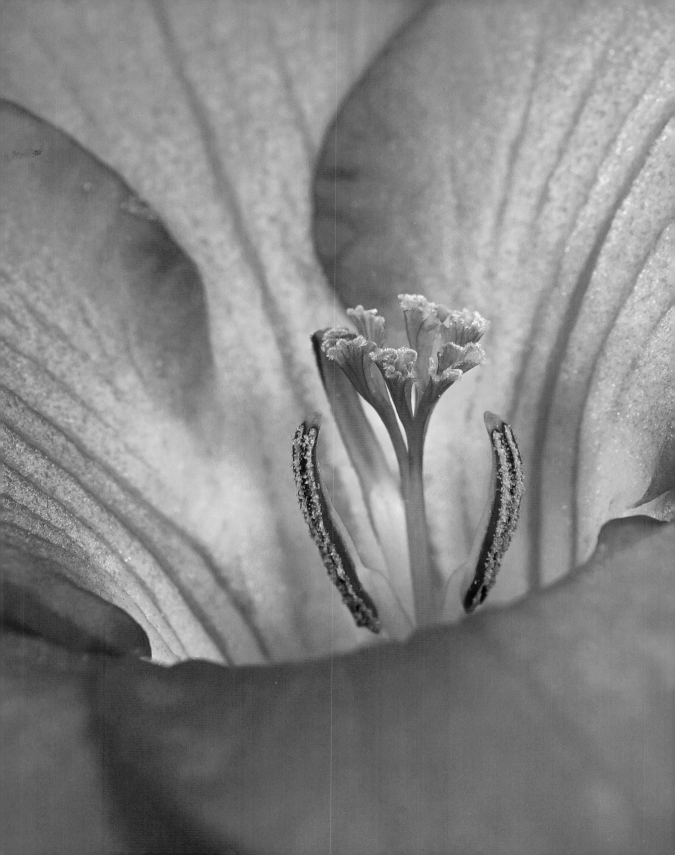

Adding the Tantric Element

The Orgasm Loop integrates this creative visualization with Tantra, Eastern lovemaking arts, to take advantage of a woman's natural sexual arousal patterns. The Tantric part of the Loop integrates physical techniques such as fire breathing (deep breathing in which you imagine the breath is hot, sexual, and on fire) and muscle flexing. Physical moves include manual clitoral stimulation. The Tantric breathing technique lays a physical track for the Loop to follow.

The Orgasm Loop didn't come together, however, until one day when I was talking to an old family friend named Rick Hasamear—a man with several black belts in karate, tae kwon do, and other martial arts. It was during our conversation on these arts that I realized that energy focus as practiced by the experts is the real key to the Loop's success.

We all possess a great deal of energy—mental, emotional, and physical. Unless they practice martial arts or kundalini (sexual) yoga, most people have no idea how much erotic energy they have or how to use it. The energy focuses utilized by martial arts experts and kundalini devotees are not so different from each other, except that martial artists focus on their chi, a spot below the navel they consider the energy source, while kundalini practitioners see their energy as primarily sexual and coiled like a serpent at the base of their spines.

Through a series of physical and mental exercises, kundalini aims to achieve three basic goals: to develop mental focus, to visualize energy movement, and to increase awareness or consciousness of the sexual energy suffusing the body and spirit. Although the energy is used for different purposes—like smashing concrete blocks or self-defense—the various martial arts disciplines have the same basic goals: to focus, visualize, and move energy. Once the yogi or the black belt concentrates, he or she feels the heat either below the navel (the chi) or in the lower back (the seat of kundalini energy). The Orgasm Loop puts both sites of energy to good use, because awakening and moving that energy into the genitals generates sexual arousal.

When you start focusing on that energy in your body, you will feel it—*and* you'll be able to control it.

What the Research Says

YOU CAN SEE ENERGY!

A 2003 British study of aikido practitioners showed that the energy in their hands immediately following a demonstration of martial arts could be measured. Thermographic (heat-seeking) video cameras scanned the practitioners' palms and recorded that their body temperatures rose by as much as four or five degrees above the temperatures recorded in their palms before the aikido activities. Their energy glowed in the photos the camera captured.

Real Talk

"I used a vasodilator, a little suction cup that you put over your clitoris before you have sex. It makes that little thing stand up more. I did feel my clitoris more… but no O. Besides, it is annoying to use and not all that comfortable."

—Charlene, 38

"My doctor prescribed testosterone cream. It does make me hornier. It doesn't make me orgasm during intercourse alone."

—Jill, 42

"Sometimes I go into the bathroom and masturbate to a high arousal level, then come out and seduce my husband. If he moves fast enough, I can come this way."

—Kerri, 32

"Dream Cream. You rub it into your clitoris and surrounding area. It really does increase sensitivity and did help me get an intercourse orgasm a few times. But don't buy cheap creams or gels in those cheap sex toy shops. I did and got an allergic rash."

—Dominique, 34

And So the Orgasm Loop Was Created

I knew I had all the pieces together with the addition of energy focus. Since I began teaching women my Orgasm Loop techniques four years ago, more than 500 women have successfully used the Loop. More than 75 percent can reach orgasm during intercourse *without touching themselves* by using the Loop.

Please understand that the "no touching" rule some women apply when using the Loop is self-imposed. It's their idea, not mine. The most natural and easiest thing to do to have an orgasm during intercourse is to give yourself the clitoral stimulation you need while he is thrusting. And a lot of men like that because they like to watch.

The Orgasm Loop works because it makes you aware of your own arousal, increases that arousal, and intensifies it so that orgasm is as inevitable for you as it is for him. It works with no hands. But there's never anything wrong with giving yourself a helping hand.

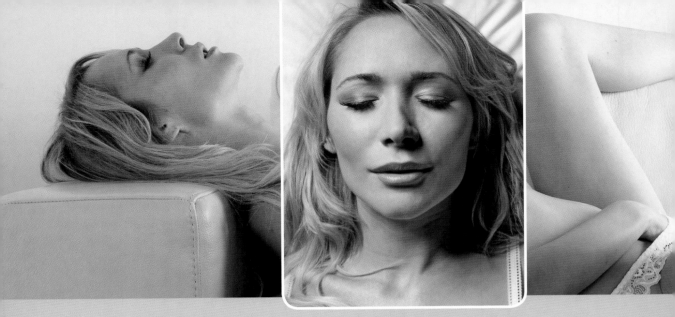

Chapter 2

How the O Loop Works

"When a woman sees a strong sexual image, her body is primed for sex before the mind has a chance to talk her out of arousal. If she loses the image before she feels arousal, the sex-negative mind has won."

—Dr. Ellen Laan, University of Amsterdam sex researcher

TODAY'S WOMAN SUFFERS from the tyranny of the "toos"—too busy, too tired, too distracted, too mad at him, feeling too fat for sex, and, of course, comparing herself too often to all of those size-two models and actresses: an exercise that doesn't boost the average female libido.

Women complain that they have trouble becoming aroused or sustaining arousal in lovemaking because of these issues. That arousal problem compounds their orgasm difficulties. How do you get to orgasm if you can't get into arousal?

Why do women find so many excuses for not getting aroused? Recent trial studies conducted by the large drug companies, including Pfizer, the makers of Viagra, have strengthened the conclusion—that anyone who's interviewed women about their sex lives already reached some time ago—that much of a woman's difficulty with sex is mental. There is no female Viagra because women's arousal issues aren't as simple as men's: increasing blood flow to the penis. If she doesn't get into a sexual mind-set, orgasm might not happen for her. And she needs to get there fast or sex takes too long.

You know the physical issue: most women don't reach orgasm via the friction from intercourse alone, and they don't like to take the direct route of using their hand to give themselves additional clitoral stimulation.

The Orgasm Loop starts where the trouble begins: in your head.

The Orgasm Loop, Step by Step

In this chapter you'll learn the three-step Orgasm Loop technique that will change your sex life. Don't hurry. Take your time learning each step. This is your path to reliable orgasms. There's no need to rush.

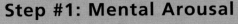

Step #1: Mental Arousal

Close your eyes, clear your mind of distractions, and visualize your own arousal.

Some women, for instance, might visualize their genitalia—lips swelling, moisture forming, the color changing to deeper pink. Other women might visualize a flower, perhaps an orchid. (The sensual flower paintings of Georgia O'Keefe can be an inspiration. See page 21.) Some women might see arousal as a color, perhaps pink, red, or saffron yellow, the color of Saraswati, the Hindu goddess of knowledge and the arts, who embodies the wisdom of Devi, mother goddess in Hindu mythology. A beach at sunset can be an arousal image, too.

Find the image that represents arousal to you and focus on it every time you use the Orgasm Loop. This image must become your mental equivalent of an erotic mantra. Focus to the extent that no other image enters your mind.

What the Research Says

AROUSAL PRECEDES DESIRE

For decades sex researchers and therapists accepted the model of sexual response developed in the 1960s by the grandparents of sex therapy, Dr. William Masters and Dr. Virginia Johnson: desire precedes arousal.

New studies contradict that. Neurobiologists report that women's brains are blazing with arousal before they even experience desire for a sexual encounter. A 2005 University of Amsterdam study, for example, demonstrated that a woman's arousal is triggered almost instantly by sexual imagery.

Show a woman the right sexy image and her body responds before she has even begun to think about wanting sex.

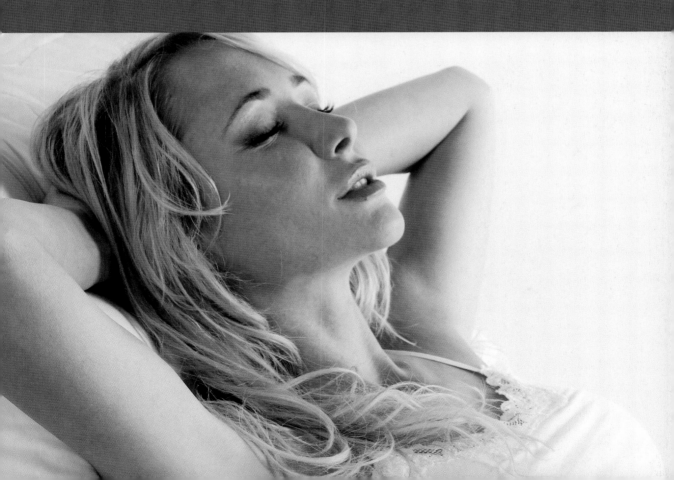

THE AROUSAL IMAGE CANNOT BE YOUR LOVER

The secret to choosing an arousal image is keeping the image simple, clean, and constant so that every time you see it in your mind, you think: I am aroused. The more you use the image, the more you condition yourself to be aroused. But it can't be a mental photo of your partner.

The image of the one you love might call up different emotions depending on whether or not he (or she) did his share of the chores that week or any number of other factors. Our ideas and outlooks on our husbands/partners change so much from day to day, and our feelings about them aren't always positive. All of those changes are bound to sabotage our arousal image if theirs is the image we're using. And even though we love them, our partners should not own our arousal. After all, we don't own theirs. (Remember that old saying, "Men share themselves with women; women give themselves to men"?)

You need to tap into arousal as a pure force of its own volition—a force inside you—not a complicated, varied emotion dependent on your partner. Love is complex. Arousal is simple. The O Loop lets you get inside your own sexual moment.

Real Talk

"My body! I gained weight with two pregnancies and didn't lose
it all. Even if I could take off the extra twenty pounds I'm carrying,
I wouldn't look like I did when he married me. I have stretch
marks. My breasts aren't perky anymore. I used to love my body
and sex was good."

—Melanie, 34

"Anything! Everything! I am a control freak and I can't let go until
everything is done. When is everything ever done?"

—Gail, 44

"Am I going to see this guy again? I've had two relationships end
with the guy not calling anymore after a few months. Maybe I'm
not sexy enough to keep a man."

—Angela, 23

Step #2: Energy Focus

When you are conscious of nothing but arousal, turn your focus inward toward your energy sites.

First, focus on the spot just below your navel (the inner chi). Breath deeply and slowly and imagine that little spot of energy glowing and growing. Move it down into your genitals with your mind.

Hold that energy in place.

Next, imagine a fiery coil of sexual energy (kundalini) located at the base of your spine. Uncoil it and move it into your genitals. Feel the undulating energy as it uncoils and circles around and through the spot of glowing energy you've already moved down.

Now you have moved your body's energy into your genitals. Your clitoris is on fire with it. And you are experiencing heightened sensitivity to touch because you have created a physiological response in your body simply by using your consciousness. Your heartbeat is accelerated. Your body temperature is rising. You feel more alive, more sensuous with the heat. And the blood flow concentrated in your genitals is making them incredibly sensitive.

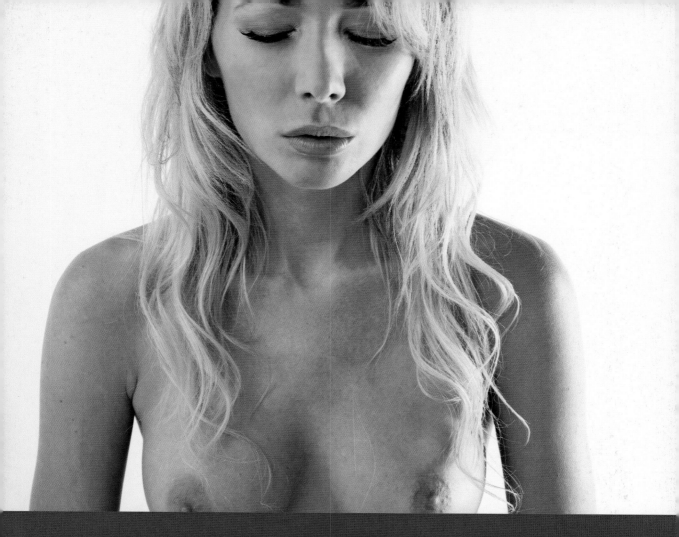

LEARN HOW TO SEE ENERGY

Energy focus is a new concept for the Western mind. Easterners are comfortable with the idea of moving that energy within the body.

Try something that karate instructors teach beginners. Stretch one arm out in front of your body, fingers spread and palm down. Imagine that you are pressing down against a strong force. Will your hand to stay level while keeping that force in place. Feel your palm getting warmer? (If not, try again later.) That is the force of the energy you moved into your hand.

Now press your warm hand against your genitals. Do you feel the heat?

You can move that heat into your genitals through energy focus alone.

#3

Step #3: Physical Moves

While maintaining your energy focus, use fire breathing to intensify the mind/genital connection. Imagine you are breathing fire in a circle, inhaling it up from your genitals throughout your body and exhaling it out your mouth. Envision that erotic fire as a circle. Keep the fire going in a circular fashion.

Once you have created a circle of fire, flex your PC muscles (see below) in time with your breathing. Tighten them as you breathe in; loosen them as you breathe out. The combination of controlled breathing

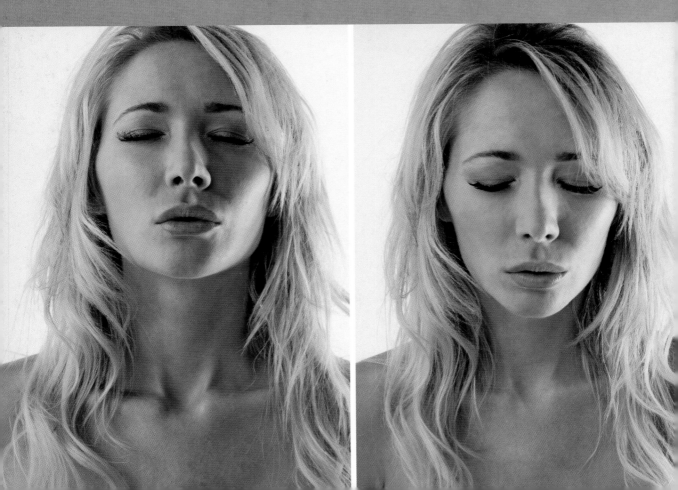

and energy focusing creates a lot of heat. You literally move that heat in and out of your body. Like any form of deep breathing, fire breathing increases the oxygen level in the blood. And it forces more blood into your genital area.

Keep up the fire breathing during intercourse. Don't worry if you lose a cycle or two. Just pick it up again, especially at the point of orgasm, because fire breathing intensifies orgasm.

Apply clitoral stimulation if you need it or simply want it. But you probably won't need a lot of additional stimulation to achieve orgasm if you've been following these steps!

"**Orgasm can be more** a mental response than a physical one. Feeling badly about yourself and your sexuality—and concentrating on those feelings—can be a self-fulfilling prophecy. A positive sexual image is so important."

—Yvonne K. Fulbright, sex educator and author of
Touch Me There!: A Hands-On Guide to Your Orgasmic Hot Spots

HOW IMPORTANT IS A STRONG PC (PUBOCOCCYGEUS) MUSCLE IN ACHIEVING ORGASM? VERY!

Kegel exercises are the key to a great sex life. A strong pubococcygeus (PC) muscle makes orgasm more likely, and more intense. It also facilitates multiple or extended orgasms. And it keeps the vagina toned after childbirth, even after menopause.

The PC muscle is a hammock-like muscle that stretches from the pubic bone to the coccyx (tailbone) in both sexes. It forms the floor of your pelvic cavity. Locate your PC muscle by stopping and starting the flow of urine.

While you're working on your energy focus and breathing techniques, try working on your PC muscle tone as well. Start with:

A SHORT KEGEL SEQUENCE. Contract the muscle twenty times at approximately one squeeze per second. Exhale gently as you tighten only the muscles around your genitals (including the anus), but not the muscles in your buttocks. Don't bear down when you release. Simply let go.

Do two sessions twice a day. Gradually build up to two sets of seventy-five per day.

Then add:

A LONG KEGEL SEQUENCE. Hold the muscle contractions for a count of three. Relax between contractions. Work up to holding for ten seconds, and then relaxing for ten seconds. Again, start with two sets of twenty each and build up to seventy-five.

At this point you will be doing three hundred sets a day of the combined short and long sequences. Next, be ready to add:

THE PUSH-OUT. After releasing the contraction, push down and out gently, as if you were having a bowel movement with your PC muscle. I said *gently*.

Once you've mastered the push-out, create Kegel sequences that combine long and short repetitions with push-outs. After six weeks of daily sets of three hundred, you should have a well-developed PC and you can keep it that way by doing a hundred and fifty sets several times a week.

RAISE YOUR KEGEL

Laura Berman, Ph.D., sex therapist, and director of the Berman Center in Chicago (and frequent *Oprah* guest), suggests this advanced Kegel variation to spice up the routine:

Lie on your back, with your legs straight.

Do a Kegel and hold the contraction as you pull in your stomach.

Still holding the contraction, raise one leg, forming a right angle to your body. Open your leg wide to the right, return to center, then cross your leg to the left of your body.

Release the contraction.

Repeat with your other leg.

Do three sets of ten with each leg.

POWER KEGELS

"Dr. Arnold Kegel originally designed his exercises for use with a resistance device to ensure their effectiveness," says Howard Glazer, Ph.D., a psychologist who specializes in pelvic-floor muscle diagnosis and rehabilitation.

He has his patients use the Kegelmaster 2000, a salad tong–like tool that tones the PC muscle by using resistance. Here's how it works: You insert the open end of the Kegelmaster 2000 into your vagina. Then you contract and release the PC muscle, which closes and opens the tool.

Kegel barbells work on the same principle, but you pull them into your vagina on the contraction and push them out on the release. (You can order barbells from babeland.com and candidaroyalle.com.)

Glazer says that the typical "five minutes or less" Kegel workout isn't enough. He prescribes a ten-second hold followed by a ten-second rest, repeated sixty times over twenty minutes, twice a day for six to eight weeks, with ongoing biweekly sessions thereafter.

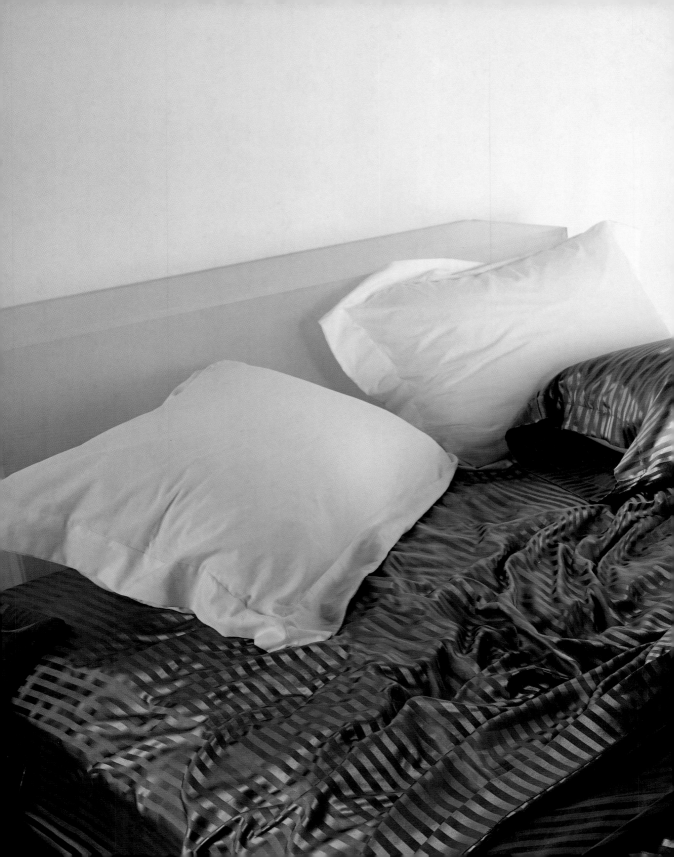

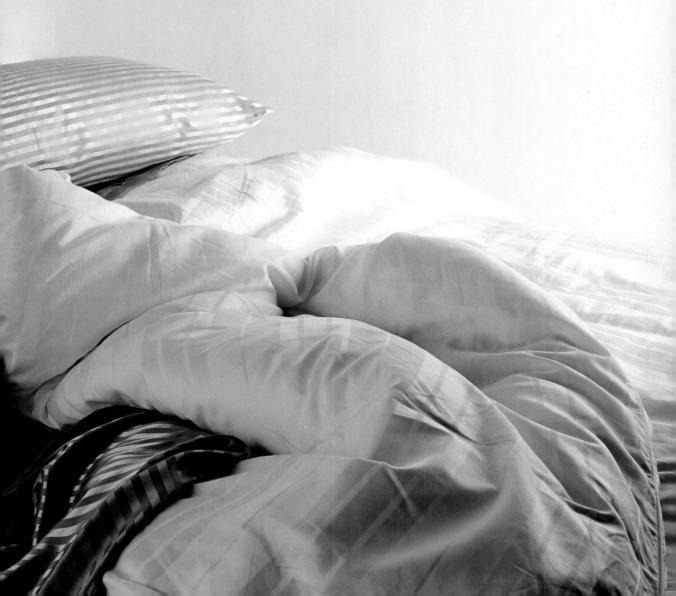

Part 2

The O Loop for Beginners

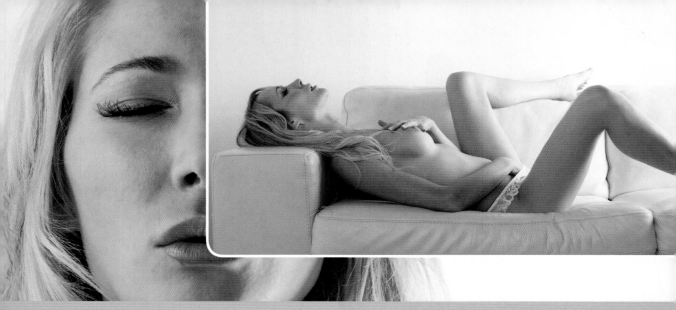

Step 1

Use the O Loop to Achieve Orgasm Solo

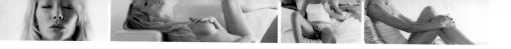

WOMEN MASTURBATED before the 1970s, but they didn't learn how to do it from a book.

Dr. Lonnie Barbach's 1975 landmark sex book *For Yourself*, which baby boomer mothers handed to their daughters, was the best-selling gentle guide to sexual self-discovery that said to women, in a nutshell, "Honey, it's okay to masturbate; you have to learn how your body works so you'll be ready to have good sex with him." In 1986, another book, *Sex for One*, by Betty Dodson, the "grandmother of masturbation," redefined the cultural mind-set on female masturbation. Dodson dared to say, in effect, "Ladies, you are entitled to orgasm, and masturbation might be the only way you ever get one." It was a masturbation and orgasm manifesto!

These two books brought masturbation out of the dark while simultaneously launching the orgasm book industry. These guides were not only aimed at helping women reach orgasm, preferably during sexual intercourse, but they were also intending to teach women how to have longer, bigger, stronger, extended, expanded orgasms—superlatives not so likely for most women. The Orgasm Loop takes orgasm advice into the twenty-first century, where we finally lay to rest the misconception that women don't care about orgasm and acknowledge that a root cause of low desire is the difficulty women have in reaching orgasm. You can use the Loop with your lover, whether male or female, though for the sake of simplicity, I'm calling that other person "him."

But first you need to use the Loop by yourself in tandem with masturbation. Doing so will enable you to learn how your own arousal patterns work, without outside pressure from your partner.

Women who rarely (or never) experience orgasm will spend more time on this exercise. If reaching orgasm is highly problematic for you, don't use the O Loop with your partner until you've had *ten* orgasms alone.

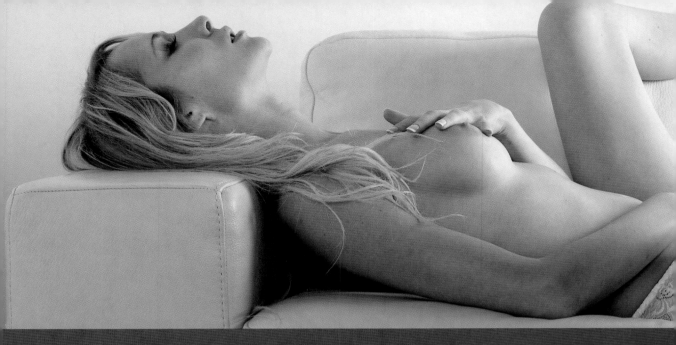

What the Research Says

HOW MANY WOMEN MASTURBATE?

Various statistics put the percentage of women who masturbate anywhere from 60 to 90 percent. In 1953, Kinsey reported that 62 percent of women he surveyed did masturbate, with 53 percent reaching orgasm that way. Then in 1974 sexologist Shere Hite reported in her massive survey of female sexual behavior and attitudes, *The Hite Report*, that two-thirds of women surveyed masturbated, with 90 percent of them reaching orgasm.

Interestingly, a 2004 Toronto study found that 55 percent of women begin masturbating in their teens, but almost half stop when they are in monogamous relationships, especially marriage. Yet 81 percent of men continue to masturbate while in relationships. Why do men and women differ so greatly here? As much as they love us—and they do love us—men separate love and sex. If they are aroused and want quick release, they masturbate. And they don't consider it "cheating" on the relationship.

Women, on the other hand, tie their sexuality into their relationships. Either they feel guilty if they take pleasure in masturbating or they fear something is wrong in the relationship if it doesn't meet all of their sexual needs. Realistically, we all want and need to masturbate sometimes. But women tend to squash the parts of their sexuality that don't conform to the prevailing model of behavior.

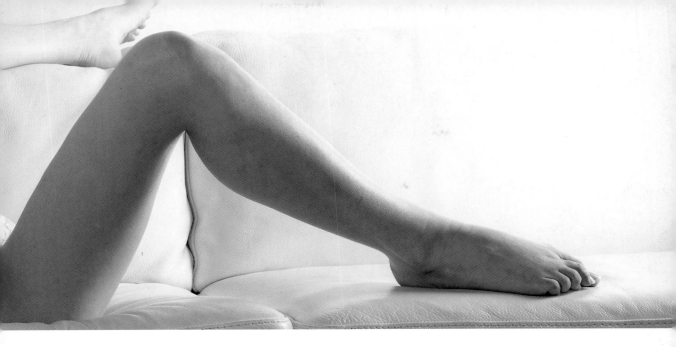

Why Masturbate?

Why not go straight to using the Orgasm Loop during intercourse? Because you need the time alone to master the technique. If you're paying attention to your partner's needs and responses the first few times you use the O Loop, you won't be able to do the one thing you must do—focus on yourself.

There are three key reasons to use the O Loop with masturbation first:

1. **While the Orgasm Loop is simple and easy to use once you have learned it, you will learn it better on your own.**

   When you are masturbating, you're focused solely on your own pleasure. No distractions. You have the same effective mind-body connection that men always have during masturbation and lovemaking. Their external genitals give them an advantage in reaching orgasm because they physically see their sexual arousal. Women, however, can learn to do what men do naturally. Especially if you only rarely reach orgasm, you need the private space where this mind-body connection is solid to begin making orgasm happen on a reliable basis.

2. **You experience orgasm more intensely during masturbation than during lovemaking.**

   Yes, that is true for women and men. Orgasm during masturbation is a mainly physical event (with mental and emotional benefits). In lovemaking—especially for women—it is a more complex physical, emotional, and psychological event. That complexity inevitably makes us experience the orgasm in a more diffuse way. I am not denigrating the joys of partner sex and the orgasms found there. But an orgasm experienced alone is not influenced by emotional connection. It is pure, and it is all yours.

3. **Masturbation is good for you.**

And it's not sex's stepsister. It's a vital part of your sex life. Hopefully, you will be masturbating to the O Loop even after you have taken it out to partner play. Masturbating to orgasm aids cardiovascular health, relieves tension, stimulates your imagination, keeps you sexually viable during celibate periods, and can relieve depression and boost self-esteem. And no matter what you heard from Mom, the church, or backward gal pals, there is no credible evidence of mental or physical ill effects from masturbation. Female sexual empowerment is and long has been an intimidating concept in our society. And what is more empowering than controlling your own orgasm?

Another big plus: masturbation takes the pressure off your relationship. When your orgasm doesn't depend on another, you can relax and enjoy lovemaking. Lonnie Barbach (internationally renowned psychologist and sex therapist) was right. Masturbation is absolutely *necessary* for a woman to learn how she becomes aroused and reaches orgasm. And it is much more than that: it is sexual empowerment of the kind that men are born into.

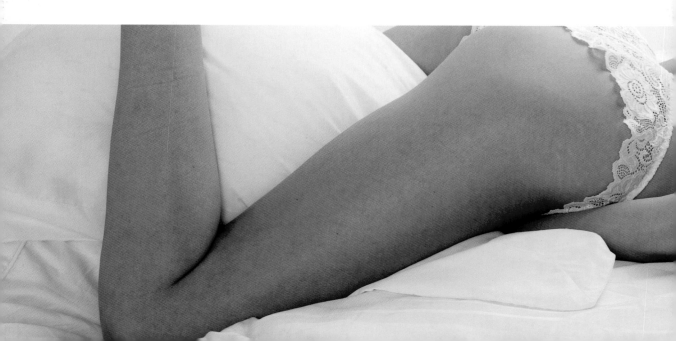

What the Research Says

COMMON WAYS FEMALES MASTURBATE

Based on my own research and interviews, *Cosmopolitan* magazine surveys, and research provided by Dr. Patti Britton, the most common ways that women masturbate are:

- Stroking or rubbing the clitoris and surrounding area with a hand and/or vibrator.

- Inserting fingers (or a vibrator) into the vagina to stimulate the G-spot, the rough patch of skin partway up the vaginal canal. (For more on stimulating the G-spot, and other his-and-hers hot spots, see Chapter 4.)

- Directing the flow of water to the genitals in the tub or shower.

- Lying face down on the bed, usually straddling a pillow, and rubbing against the pillow or mattress.

- Standing up and rubbing against a hard surface, for example, the corner of a dresser or nightstand.

- Crossing the legs tightly and clenching them together while flexing the PC muscle.

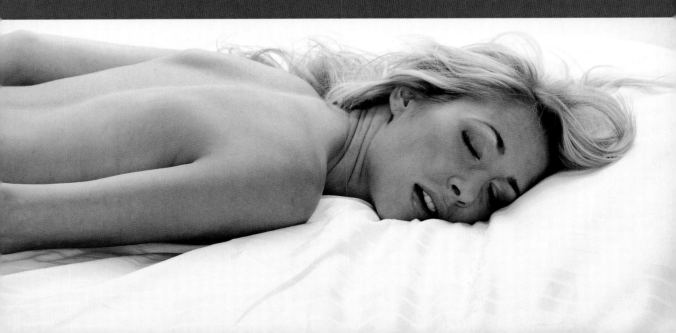

FIRST, YOU MUST COME

If you have never experienced orgasm, buy a vibrator. Why? Because if you seldom masturbate or you don't manually stimulate yourself to reach orgasm during intercourse, that probably means you aren't comfortable using your hands. (Otherwise, you would have put them to use already.) You will also be more likely to put the time into learning the O Loop if you know how good orgasm feels. Play with that vibe until you do come.

The best vibrators for virgins are external vibes, not meant for insertion. Many women equate "sex" with insertion, but insertion—like intercourse alone—doesn't bring the majority of women to orgasm. Use an external vibe to stimulate your clitoris and surrounding area directly—it's the *fastest* route to orgasm for nearly every woman.

Start with the lowest speed applied in a circular fashion around the clitoris. You can increase speed and clitoral contact as desired.

Some good external vibes include:

- The Hitachi Magic Wand, so big and powerful that many women can reach orgasm in seconds.

- Laya Spot or Chandra, small clitoral vibes.

- Shower vibes like the Ducky vibe—shaped like your rubber ducky from childhood—or the Water Shimmer.

For more information on vibes, see Step 2 (page 52).

What the Research Says

REACHING ORGASM TAKES TIME

Studies show that women reach orgasm via masturbation as easily as men do. How long does it take? Thirty seconds to five minutes, with the average being four minutes. Women who masturbate to multiples can spend many more minutes in orgasm.

Break the Orgasm Loop Down into Components— and Master Them

Spend at least three and up to ten days of daily practice in gaining mastery of the Orgasm Loop components. This need not take more than thirty minutes a day, unless you want to spend more time practicing. Women who tested the technique reported more early success when they did not need to break their concentration and refer to the book to remember "what's next."

These are the major components of the O Loop:

1. **Flirt with arousal.**

   Pick your arousal image as outlined in the Orgasm Loop technique in Chapter 2. Tape it to the refrigerator, inside your closet door, or another place where you will see it frequently. Frame it, if that's possible, and hang it on the wall in your bedroom. Live with that image for a few days before you take it (mentally) to bed. Whenever you glance at your arousal image, feel desire. Now close your eyes and see that image in your mind and feel it arousing you.

2. **Practice your Kegels daily.**

   Do the Kegel exercises introduced in Chapter 2. This is the one essential exercise that no woman can afford to ignore. The sets are quick and easy and provide many benefits, from stronger orgasms to avoiding incontinence associated with age. Your PC muscle is critical! Every time you do a Kegel set, think: this is turning me on. Associate Kegels with arousal in your mind and your body will follow.

3. **Practice fire breathing daily.**

   While lying in bed or on the couch, do the fire breathing exercise explained in Chapter 2 until you feel very aroused. Add the PC flex in time with your breathing.

4. **Move that energy!**

   For many women, the most challenging part of the Orgasm Loop is energy focus, also introduced in Chapter 2. The concept is difficult to comprehend for those who haven't studied yoga, Tantra, or martial arts, but it is not difficult to do. And it is the key to making the Orgasm Loop more than another tip for boosting orgasm. Feel that energy beginning as a spot (chi) below your navel, a snake tightly curled at the base of your spine. Focus on the energy and make it grow and spread into your genitals.

"**I had an orgasm** in the gym lifting weights, but I was doing Kegels at the time. It was probably the Kegels."

—Carmen Diaz, American actress and former fashion model

Real Talk

"I picked a Georgia O'Keefe flower print that I have always loved—'Red Canna.' Her flower paintings are so erotic. And the color red puts it over the top for me. I just look at that print and lubricate, so I was into my arousal image immediately."

—Kim, 35

"The mental imaging didn't come easily for me. I picked a color, hot pink, and discarded that. A photo of sand dunes was appealing, but I settled on a swatch of fabric printed with a leopard-skin pattern. That worked for me."

—Maggie, 42

"I thought it would be the ocean, but I found myself hearing the waves when I looked at the photo. Colors and flowers made me restless. Van Gogh's 'Starry Night' was finally the choice. It is soothing and disturbing all at once, and I find that arousing."

—Pia, 29

Put It All Together

Some women like a little romance when they masturbate. Fragrance, flowers, and the best sheets are all fine as long as they enhance rather than detract from your experience. Even soft music and candlelight might distract you. In the beginning, anything might distract you. So pare down. Once you have mastered the O Loop, you can add whatever sensual and erotic elements you like. For starters, however, keep it simple.

Get into a comfortable position, for example, reclining on your back with knees bent, feet on the bed. That classic position takes the stress off your back and gives you easy access to stimulating your clitoris and vagina. Any masturbation or intercourse position you favor is good. Find what works for you.

As directed in Chapter 2, practice the Orgasm Loop:

1. **Meditate on your arousal image.** As you focus on arousal, your nipples might grow erect, your pulse rate will increase, and your genitals will lubricate.

2. **Focus your sexual energy into your genitals.** Imagine that energy moving from your chi and the small of your back and turning into fiery desire in your genitals.

3. **Add the fire breathing and PC flexing elements of the Orgasm Loop technique.** Coordinate your circular breath of fire with PC flexing so that you contract as the fire is pulled into your body and release as it is expelled.

Then add a step:

4. **When you are highly aroused, use your hand or a vibrator to bring you to orgasm.** (More detailed instructions on vibrators in the next chapter!)

You don't have to be a no-hands purist to use the Orgasm Loop, even in partner sex. If you feel agonizingly close to orgasm and crave direct clitoral stimulation to get there—touch yourself. Or pick up the small vibe you should always keep conveniently nearby. Some women will be orgasmic from the O Loop alone; some women will always need a little direct stimulation to finish.

And Repeat

Continue masturbating to multiple orgasms using the O Loop. Multiple orgasms should not seem like a goal you have to reach. This is sex, not the New York City marathon. But, in fact, most women can have multiple orgasms if they continue the stimulation through their orgasm and don't let their arousal subside. So try it for the pleasure.

Real Talk

WAS IT GOOD FOR YOU?

"I'd had exactly two orgasms in my whole life before I learned how to do the O Loop. When I was in college, I used a vibrator until I was chafed—and did not come! [With the O Loop] the breathing and flexing and energy focusing really get me high. From there it only takes a little bit of vibe play to put me over."

—Jamie, 32

"Yes, it has put me in control. And I love that! I know how to come now."

—Kristin, 29

"Orgasms are really difficult for me. But this is helping. I am still working on making my ten masturbation orgasms before I take the O Loop out for a run with the boyfriend."

—Chandra, 36

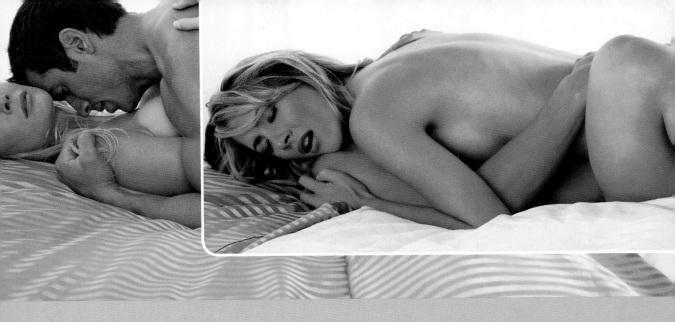

Step 2

Bridge Solo Sex and Partner Sex by Adding the Vibe

"Vibrators provide one of the most consistent and strongest forms of stimulation. For a lot of gals, they remove that nagging doubt: Will I come or not?"

—Dr. Judy Kuriansky, sex therapist and author of *Generation Sex: America's Hottest Sex Therapist Answers the Hottest Questions About Sex*

UP TO THIS POINT, you might have used a vibrator (or touched yourself) to reach orgasm while you were mastering the Orgasm Loop because you needed the additional clitoral stimulation to reach orgasm. Now incorporate vibe play *into* the O Loop, whether or not you need this direct clitoral stimulation to come. Use the vibe as a separate activity.

Here's why:

- Vibrator play is a bridge activity between masturbation and partner sex. Using the vibe will help you learn how to incorporate other erotic activities into the O Loop without losing your focus. Unlike a lover, the vibe is completely under your control. If it gets too distracting, you can switch it off.

- Vibrators are sex-life enhancement aides. They help you create new physical sensations. With so many styles, shapes, and sizes of vibrators on the market, there is one for every woman's every mood. If you have never experienced a G-spot orgasm or multiple orgasms, you probably will do so with a vibe.

- Contrary to myth, you won't become "dependent" on a vibrator for orgasm, especially using the O Loop. But having a vibe at your disposal is reassuring. You know that you can pick one up and have an orgasm even if you do lose your focus during sex with your partner now and then.

- Sometimes you may want to use a vibrator to kick-start the Orgasm Loop. If you are particularly stressed, a few preliminary minutes (or seconds) with the vibrator can take the edge off. Use the vibe until you are aware of arousal, and then you can get into your arousal image.

The Vibrator Shopping Guide

If you don't own a vibrator, it's time to go shopping. And if you do have one or two vibrators, check out the irresistible new high-tech toys. No sex toy shops or parties in your neighborhood? There are excellent online sources for vibes, lubes, and all sorts of toys. My favorite is Babeland.com, which is owned by two fabulous women, for its range of sex toys, the user-friendliness of the site, the frequent sales and specials, and the helpful information.

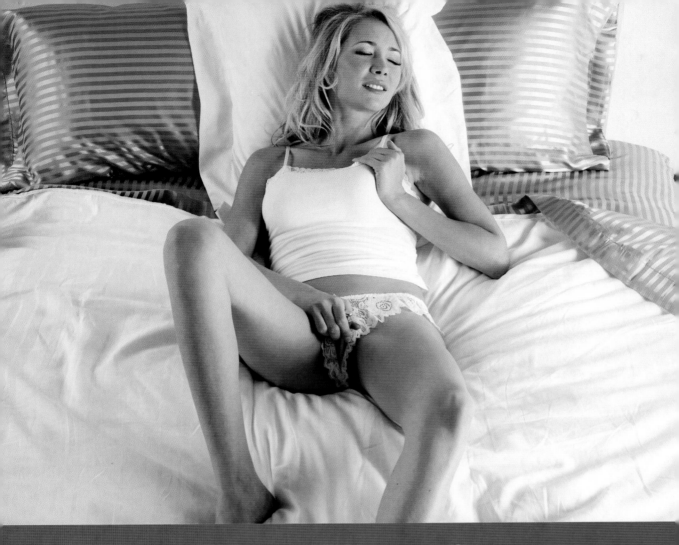

What the Research Says

WOMEN ARE IN A MASTURBATION RUT

Sex researcher Shere Hite states in her survey of female sexual behavior and attitudes, *The Hite Report*, that only 11 percent of women use more than one method of masturbation. That means the overwhelming majority of women are, according to Hite, treating masturbation like the "quickest route to orgasm" instead of "an exploratory exercise." Vibrators, she suggests, can help women "branch out."

Most women use the method that worked when they first started masturbating as teenagers.

The majority of vibrators are designed to stimulate the clitoris and are used externally. Some go inside, like dildos, and simulate the penile thrusting of intercourse. Others are waterproof so you can use them in the bath, shower, hot tub, or pool. There are even remote-controlled vibrators that your lover can control.

To the women who love them, shopping for vibes is as fun as shopping for shoes.

The Classic External Vibes

External vibes are either oversized or contour-shaped to fit the way your body curves, and they get the job done.

Hitachi Magic Wand

Labeled "a sex toy that changed the world" by Babeland.com, Hitachi is perhaps the largest selling vibrator in the world. A very large and powerful vibrator, it is marketed as "a muscle massager" and is available in drugstores as well as sex toy shops. And, wow, does it make those muscles vibrate!

You might want to keep your panties on if you're using the Hitachi. The vibrations, even on low speed, can be quite intense. A little piece of cloth can prevent chafing.

Eroscillator 2

The only sex toy endorsed by legendary Dr. Ruth Westheimer, the Eroscillator resembles an electric toothbrush in size and shape. It "eroscillates," or moves back and forth, rather than vibrates, so the motion is more gentle against the clitoris, but still effective.

Pocket Rocket 1

Tiny but relatively powerful compared to its size, this one tucks away into a small handbag and gets the job done anywhere, anytime. You can change the texture of the vibe and the feeling of the vibrations by adding a "jelly" sleeve, a soft covering with little nubs that stimulate the clitoris.

Water Dancer

This is the waterproof version of the Pocket Rocket—it's great for combining the morning shower with the first orgasm of the day.

Finger Vibes, such as Fukuoku 9000

The top-of-the-line finger vibe, Fukuoku, is a great couple's toy. Finger vibes wrap around your finger or fit over it and are perfect for clitoral stimulation during intercourse. Finger Fun is a slightly larger, waterproof version.

Strap-on Vibes, such as the Butterfly
A strap-on vibrator stimulates her clitoris during intercourse while giving him pleasurable sensations, too. The Sweetheart and many other vibes, some remote-controlled, work the same way as the Butterfly.

The Classic Internal Vibes
Internal vibes are inserted into your vagina and simulate intercourse.

The Rabbit (with Pearls)
The Rabbit stimulates three erogenous zones at once. In addition to G-spot stimulation, the ears of the rabbit riding the shaft tickle your clitoris, and the vibrating band of pearls around the base stimulates your vaginal opening. Some rabbits come without the pearls, but the pearls are always a good idea. Why stop at two sensations when you can have three?

Try inserting the vibrating shaft so it hits your G-spot. The G-spot is a rough patch of skin roughly a third of the way up the front vaginal wall. You can find it by putting your hand to your vagina, palm up, inserting two fingers, and making the "come hither" gesture, or by using a G-spot vibe or a vibe with a G-spot attachment.

For more intense clitoral stimulation from the rabbit ears, try riding your rabbit in the female superior position. You'll smash his rubbery ears

ADD AN EXTERNAL VIBE TO THE O LOOP
Here's how to incorporate an external vibe into the O Loop:

1. Select the vibe that feels most comfortable to you in the moment. Any external vibe—from the big Hitachi to the tiny Pocket Rocket—works here. Some women find a contour vibe the best choice because it fits seamlessly between hand and body.

2. After using your arousal image, glide the vibe around your clitoris and surrounding area as you focus on energy movement.

3. Keep the vibe gliding over your clitoris and surrounding area and your vagina in time with your fire breathing and PC flexing.

4. Finally, let the vibe take you all the way to orgasm.

into your clitoris. And it's good practice for using O Loop in that position with a live partner.

G-Spot Vibes, such as the Swirl

Designed to hit the G-spot, this one and others like it are limited-use vibes. If G-spot orgasms are your thing, this is your toy. (You can also buy G-spot attachments for other vibes, including the Hitachi Magic Wand.) These vibes have angled heads to hit the G-spot easily.

Contour Vibes, such as the Laya Spot

One of the many new contour vibes, Laya is both chic and ergonomically correct. Designed to fit the curves of a woman's body, it is versatile and discreet. It fits between a woman's hand and her genitals.

Check Out the Vibe Power

Test a new vibe against the palm of your hand before using it in O Loop play. Experiment with intensity of pressure and speed. Move the vibe from your hand up your arm and around your shoulders. Caress your breasts with it. Place it against your inner thigh.

Now you know what the vibe can do.

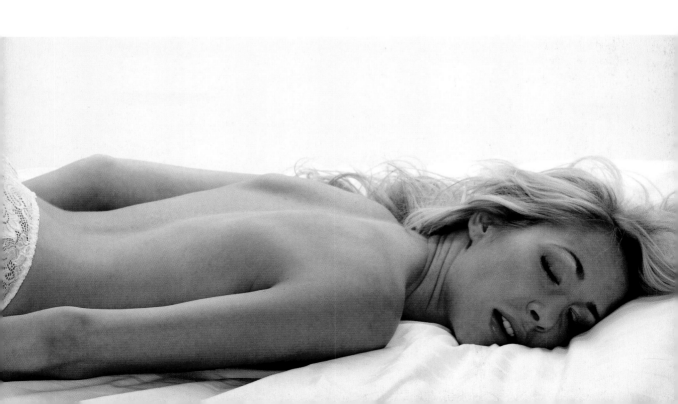

ADD AN INTERNAL VIBE TO THE ORGASM LOOP

Here's how to incorporate an internal vibe into the O Loop:

1. Pick an internal vibe that you have enjoyed before. Run it over your clitoris and the surrounding area, focusing on your arousal image and energy movement.

2. Insert the vibe and move with it in time to your fire breathing and PC flexing.

3. Ride the vibe the way you would ride his penis in any intercourse position that feels good and doesn't take your focus entirely off the O Loop. Take it to orgasm.

The New High-Tech Vibes

These high-tech vibes add sound or boost power—or both.

Talking Head

This Rabbit talks! The early (and still available) version of this interactive vibe comes with computer chips programmed to speak as "lovers," like the French man and the girl who say what you want to hear. The latest version has an MP-3 download, and you can program it within anything you like, such as your lover's voice or music. On the horizon: an alliance with Clone-a-Willy that will produce a Talking Head shaped just like your guy that speaks in his voice, too.

OhMiBod

A slim wand that connects to your iPod, this vibe puts new meaning in "feeling the music." After you program your playlist into it, the wand vibrates to your preferred beat. You can only find this one at Babeland.com.

The Cone

A big, pink, sixteen-speed cone, this one is unbelievably versatile. You can put it under you while you're kneeling on the floor performing fellatio, attach it to the wall and back into it, or put it between your legs and let it vibrate. The Cone is creative and pretty enough to leave on your night table as a piece of art.

Form 6

Dubbed "the new wonder vibe" on the Babeland.com site, Form 6 is elegant and upscale in its design and target advertising. Its name comes from its six modes and six speeds (along with five intensity levels). And it's waterproof.

Turn Off to Turn On

If you become too conscious of trying to make the vibe "work" with the O Loop, turn off the power. Focus on energy movement, fire breathing, and PC flexing. When you are into the Loop again, turn the power back on.

Putting the Vibe in Your O Loop

You've learned to use a vibrator to get yourself aroused before you even start the Orgasm Loop. And you know that you can use your vibe to help you reach orgasm when you need that direct clitoral stimulation. These are the two helping roles that a vibrator can play in the O Loop.

Now let's elevate the vibe from supporting role to star player.

Playing with vibrators can be the most fun you've had since you outgrew Barbie dolls. Vibes are brilliant. Combining vibrators with the O Loop puts you completely in charge of your orgasms. And once you feel comfortable and confident using your O Loop techniques, you can take that power into partner sex.

"How you masturbate—and how long—mirrors the type of sex you enjoy. Sensualists enjoy lengthy foreplay when they masturbate while functionalists get right down to it."

—Helen Adams, British sex researcher

Real Talk

"I use my Pocket Rocket because it seems less intrusive than other vibes. It's small yet powerful. If I am slow in getting into my arousal image, I flick it on for a minute. It's also useful at the end when I need a little help to come."

—Connie, 41

"I am in love with Form 6, and it's the only vibe I am using now. Because it has so many settings, it's the perfect vibe for every occasion. I coordinate the vibe action with my fire breathing and PC flexing. Intense!"

—Stephanie, 36

"If I am just using a vibe to help me to orgasm, I turn on the Hitachi Magic Wand. It's always under my pillow. If I'm making the vibrator part of the O Loop, I use my Rabbit. The Rabbit has it going—everywhere. Combining Rabbit play and O Loop has given me the best orgasms of my life."

—Mai, 28

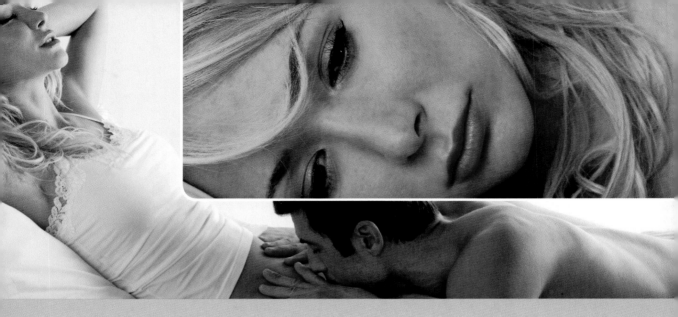

Step 3

Add a Little Help from Your Lover

"When a man loves a woman, he does what it takes to get her wherever she needs to go."

—Jay-Z, American rap artist and Beyonce's significant other

NOW THAT YOU HAVE REACHED several orgasms using the Orgasm Loop during masturbation alone and masturbation with a vibrator, you are ready to use it with your partner. If you haven't explained the O Loop to him (or her), do so before lovemaking. But there is no need to turn that little chat into a tutorial. It's not essential that your partner have anything but a rudimentary knowledge of the technique. Why? He shouldn't feel like he has to play the key role, and "give" you an orgasm. You only need his indulgence while you focus on yourself for a change. The overwhelming majority of lovers, male or female, will be happy to accommodate anything that makes your orgasm more likely rather than problematic.

But how do you explain the need for a new technique if he doesn't know you aren't having orgasms or aren't having them reliably? You can tell him the truth. "Honey, I fake more than I come." That will certainly make the case for a new approach. It might also hurt his feelings and make him angry. Some therapists and advice columnists advise telling the truth because truth telling is emotional risk taking that leads to a more intimate relationship. (Fearless truth telling is now called "radical honesty.")

However, not every relationship guru advises women to confess their history of faking. I don't. You can explain your interest in O Loop by saying, "Honey, I want to try this new orgasm technique so I can have MORE orgasms," or even "so I can be responsible for my own orgasms." No one's feelings need to get hurt. Why start something new on a low note? How empowering is that?

How to Get into Your Arousal When You're Not Alone

First, allow yourself to be selfish. Lovemaking for most women is a mutual exchange of pleasure in which each is supposed to know how to drive the other wild in bed. (At least half the women's magazine sex advice articles I've written in the past two decades ran under the cover line "How to Drive Him Wild in Bed," with the other half falling under the category "How to Tell Him What You Want.") Using the Orgasm Loop, you are breaking the "do me/I do you" pattern. You are actively taking charge of your own pleasure. Your orgasm is not dependent on what he does or doesn't do, though, ironically, you will enjoy his erotic contributions more when you aren't counting on them for orgasm. Initially, you will be more selfish in bed than you are accustomed to being. Don't feel guilty about that. Your partner won't mind.

Second, don't direct your partner. You are probably accustomed to doing so, if not verbally, then through your own method of communicating to him about what works and what doesn't. Maybe you do this by sighing happily or squirming unhappily and moving in another direction beneath his fingers or tongue. (A woman I interviewed said that in the early days of their marriage, she held her husband's ears to direct him as he performed cunnilingus. Ouch.) There's nothing wrong with communicating your sexual needs. That's a good thing. But as you adapt the O Loop to lovemaking, let go of acting as monitor and guide of your partner's technique.

Third, integrate your lover's moves into your O Loop. This is like dancing. You may be awkward the first few times you take to the floor, but gradually you pick up each another's rhythms and move together with more grace. Now you are focusing on your own arousal and not directing his moves. Yet you feel what he is doing and can respond to it without losing arousal or energy focus.

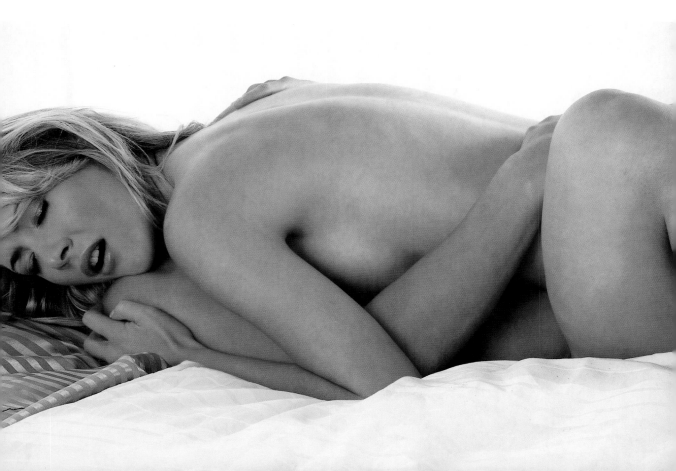

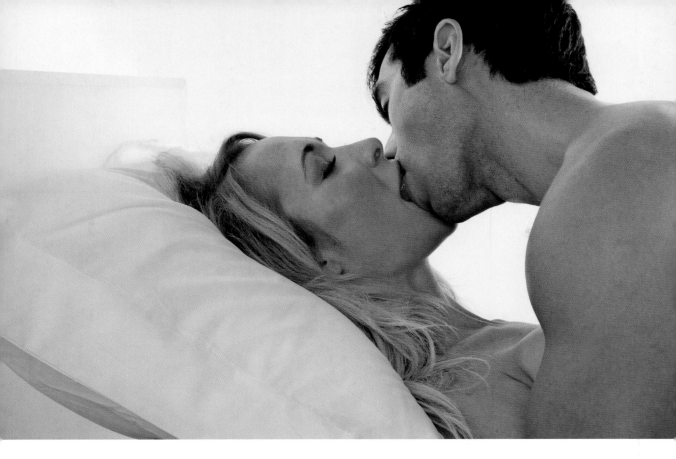

How Can You Adjust the O Loop to Lovemaking?

Sometimes a subtle change makes a big difference. That is true in everything from coloring your hair to child rearing or managing a department. And it is also true in adapting the O Loop from masturbation to lovemaking.

Here's where the little changes will occur:

1. **In the pattern of your fire breathing.**

   Kissing will naturally interrupt fire breathing. You were bringing that circle of fire into and out of your body, and suddenly there's another mouth on yours interrupting the rhythm. As you enjoy the sensations of kissing, bring that fire through your entwined mouths in time with your passionate kisses. He will feel the heat and energy, too.

   As he moves his mouth and hands over your body, return to your breathing pattern. During intercourse, adjust your fire breathing to his thrusting pattern.

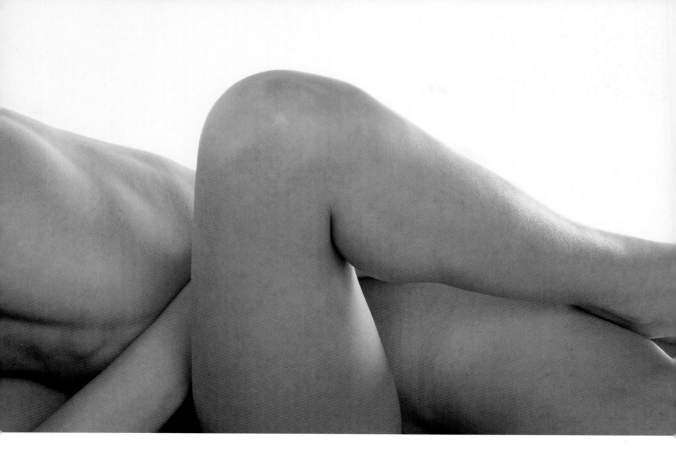

2. **In the pattern of your PC flexing pattern.**

   As he is kissing, fondling, and stroking, you might miss a few contractions and releases. Don't worry about that. Let your fire breathing guide you into picking up the pattern of flexing again.

   During intercourse, adjust your PC flexing to his thrusting pattern and your fire-breathing rhythm.

Hopefully, you will find that you don't have to concentrate hard on making these subtle changes to the O Loop. Your body, accustomed to using the Loop now, will easily shift into altered breathing and flexing modes. Gradually you will experience O Loop as more fluid—a series of moves that flow into one another—and less of a step-by-step technique.

CLOSE YOUR EYES

Eyes-wide-open sex is touted by Tantra practitioners and women's magazine writers as the most intimate way to make love. And, yes, it is rewarding. In the early days of using O Loop with your lover, however, open eyes might distract you, causing you to lose focus in both holding the arousal image mentally in place and moving your energy into your genitals.

Gazing into your lover's eyes, as with using his (or her) image for an arousal image, puts some of the power and control back into the hands of the other person. You lose touch with your own arousal. Keep your eyes closed, at least until the moment of orgasm.

When using the O Loop becomes second nature for you, then eyes open or shut won't make a difference.

Real Talk

HOW LONG DID IT TAKE YOU TO INCORPORATE THE O LOOP SUCCESSFULLY INTO LOVEMAKING?

"The third time was the charm. The first two times I lost my focus on arousal and energy moving. He was awkward and kept asking questions like, 'Is it okay if I touch your clit now?' We agreed that he wouldn't ask what he could do or verbally signal his intentions, but just make love like he would normally do. That worked. I began to experience O Loop as a seamless blend with lovemaking."

—Paula, 38

"Several times! Neither of us was comfortable with it for a while. I would start using the O Loop and he would ask me to stop doing that and 'just make love.' After a few weeks of this, I asked him to watch me masturbate using the O Loop. He was really turned on by watching me breathe heavily—and come."

—Dava, 29

But You Don't Want Your Lover to Feel "Left Out"

Admittedly, you are walking a fine line here. On the one hand, you want your lover to understand that you need to be more into yourself sexually than you normally are. On the other hand, you don't want him to feel unnecessary, like an accessory in your vibe kit.

Women who have successfully used the O Loop with their partners report that the key is making him feel a part of the process without letting him control or subvert it. So get him involved, but on your terms.

You can ask him to:

1. **Fire breathe along with you.**

   Refer him to the fire-breathing directions in Chapter 2. He can imagine his own circle of fire entering his body through his genitals and leaving through his mouth. Help him picture that breathing circle as a flaming ring of fire. Now practice fire breathing only together. Ask him to match your rhythm. (You lead, he follows.)

2. **Flex his PC muscle in time with yours or in a complementary pattern, as long as that doesn't cause you to lose focus.**

   A lot of men don't even know that they have a PC muscle in their pelvic floor! If he is one of those guys, suggest that he locate it by stopping and starting the flow of urine. Then suggest he flex that muscle when he has an erection. Watching his PC muscle influence the movement of his penis will likely inspire him to practice Kegels (see the directions for male Kegels below). Once he has gained some PC mastery, ask him to flex in time with you during intercourse.

3. **Practice energy focus as described in Chapter 2 if he is interested.**

   Men say that energy focus is the most intriguing part of the Orgasm Loop. They love hearing that it is inspired by and adapted from the martial arts. Several men told me that boxers, football players, and other athletes practice energy focus, an example being the linebacker who brings not only his weight but also his energy to bear in tackling opponents. Tell him that he can learn how to focus his body's energy into his genitals. He will be willing to try that.

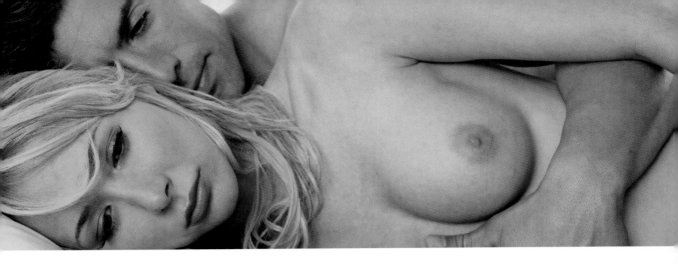

4. **Do "sexercises," exercises together that will loosen the pelvis, increase sexual flexibility, and strengthen muscles in that area.**

The exercises (scattered throughout the rest of the book) aren't a direct part of the Orgasm Loop, but they can enhance the Loop's effectiveness by improving flexibility and muscle tone in the pelvic area. Exercise also boosts production of the body's mood-enhancing chemicals. And sweating releases pheromones, the body's natural arousal scents.

Smell is the most ancient of the human senses, the one that early man relied upon for most of his information about the world around him. Recent research also backs its importance; Dr. Theresa Crenshaw's research on sex hormones, reported in 1996 in *The Alchemy of Love and Lust*, has shown that modern humans are attracted to lovers who smell "right" to us—and a little exercise brings that scent to the surface.

"Women benefit more from strengthening their PC muscles than men do. But, with a toned PC, men can experience stronger orgasms, have better ejaculatory control, and maybe firmer erections."

—Marty Klein, Ph.D., sex therapist and author of *Beyond Orgasm*

Real Talk

"Relief! He was tired of my problems reaching orgasm. Sex didn't work for me, except occasionally when it lasted for a long time. The O Loop has put me in charge. I know how to come. It's not his problem."

—Kathie, 33

"He wanted to get into it with me. He was all over the Loop, especially the fire breathing. Truthfully, that made it hard for me to work the Loop the first few times I tried it during lovemaking. But I got it together."

—Jolene, 24

"I didn't exactly tell him. I just said I was trying Tantric breathing and he thought that was cool. We haven't been together that long. I didn't want to tell him I needed a special technique to have an orgasm."

—Barbara, 50

"He said he was glad that he isn't a woman, because men just come."

—Amy, 44

SEXERCISES

Sexual yoga exercises can be both sexy and beneficial.

Why sexual yoga?

According to yoga teacher and author Jacquie Noell Greaux, these exercises are based on the five keys to good sex. That philosophy is compatible with the Orgasm Loop. The keys are: working the sexual core (abdominal, pelvic, and hip muscles), training for flexibility, controlling breathing, encouraging blood flow, and developing mind-body consciousness. Try incorporating these moves into your weekly routine:

1. **PELVIC SQUEEZES**

   Lie on your back, with your knees bent and touching, and your feet flat on the floor and also touching. Stretch out your arms above your head. Tuck your pelvis under so your back is flat against the floor. Contract your pelvic girdle muscles beneath your belly button. Lift your butt up. Squeeze your thighs together. Repeat twenty times. Do three sets of twenty two or three times a week.

2. **THE BUTT BUMP**

   Lie in the same position as above—feet and knees touching, arms outstretched overhead—but curve your back and raise your butt a few inches off the floor. Bump your butt gently to the floor three times in rapid succession. Then raise your hips off the floor and hold for three seconds. Repeat twenty times. Do three sets of twenty two or three times a week.

3. **THE BELLY ROLL**

   Lie on your back with your knees bent, your feet a few inches apart, and your arms outstretched at your sides. Lift your pelvis high so that your toes are the only part of your feet touching the floor. At the same time, raise your back so that only your shoulders are on the floor. Imagine a wave washing over your body and rolling it slowly back down to the floor, beginning in your shoulders and ending in your butt, which doesn't come all the way down. Keep the weight on your toes. Reverse the wave. Let the wave lift your body and bring it back down again in a fluid motion. Repeat twenty times. Do three sets of twenty two or three times a week.

What's Really in the O Loop for Your Lover?

Maybe you need to spell it out for him to get his full cooperation. Or maybe you simply feel compelled to make the case that your temporary selfishness is really in his best interests. Here is that case:

- Orgasm releases oxytocin, the "cuddle chemical"—the one that helps you overlook his bad habits, such as leaving his socks on the floor.

   Oxytocin makes you feel close and connected to one another. Yes, women produce more of it than men do. But the balance is more equitable after age forty. The balance becomes more equitable, incidentally, because men's oxytocin levels increase while women's oxytocin levels decrease after age forty. This is because oxytocin is also the "baby bonding" hormone, and women release a lot of it with childbirth and breastfeeding. Then, as women near the end of their prime childbearing years and hit menopause, their oxytocin levels decrease.

   Recently, some claims began surfacing in the blogosphere that Viagra increased men's oxytocin production, but that's incorrect. What Viagra actually does is enable midlife and older men to have more sex, more orgasms, and thus more opportunities for oxytocin production.

   Whatever the science behind the hormones might be, here's the bottom line: if he wants you to love him in spite of his faults, he needs to help boost your oxytocin production.

- Orgasm leads to elevation of the hormone prolactin, and orgasm during lovemaking elevates the prolactin level 400 percent more than orgasm via masturbation.

   Prolactin affects central nervous system centers controlling sexual desire. Have you heard the phrase "Sex begets sex" or "The more sex you have, the more you want to have"? Prolactin is responsible for that. It regulates dopamine, the hormone of sexual appetite.

- To ensure you get that chemical high, he needs to do what he can to help you reach orgasm reliably and often.

   And the best thing he can do is stay out of your way while you are learning to operate the Orgasm Loop during lovemaking. Suddenly the pressure is off him to "make" you come or "give" you an orgasm. He can relax and enjoy himself—and you.

- If he gets involved in fire breathing, PC flexing, and energy focus, he will reap some of the personal sexual benefits that you do from the Loop.

    He will experience his arousal more keenly. Orgasm will feel stronger to him. It might last longer. He will likely have greater control over his arousal and ejaculation. And, with his performance pressure significantly lessened, he will be able to enjoy getting into himself at the same time he's into you.

At this point, you have introduced the O Loop to your lover in a way that includes him (or her) without putting the responsibility on him to make you come. That will change the dynamic of your lovemaking in a positive way. And it will only get better as you explore the various ways to use the O Loop in your sex life together.

KEGEL EXERCISES FOR MEN

Here's how men can strengthen their PC muscle:

- First, identify your PC muscle by starting and stopping the flow of urine. That muscle can also slightly lift your erect penis when you are standing. Do your Kegels with an erection either while standing or sitting.

- Do two sets of thirty short squeezes—hold for a second, release for a second—twice a day. After a few days, add two sets of twenty long squeezes—hold and release for three seconds each. Work up to long squeezes of ten seconds each.

- Mix long and short sequences, building up to fifty sets twice a day.

Real Talk

WHAT DID HER ORGASM LOOP DO FOR YOU?

"I thought it was New Age nonsense when she first told me about it. Then I realized that she was having a good time alone with her vibrators and I wanted to get into the party. It works for her and that's a good thing for me."

—Ken, 47

"I was enthusiastic from the beginning. I know a little bit about yoga and Tantra and took tae kwon do classes as a kid, so I was into the concept. The O Loop works for her. The fire breathing and PC flexing have made sex better for me, too."

—Jason, 26

"She joked that she gave up men to become a lesbian because she never had an orgasm with a man. Truthfully, orgasm was difficult for her even with me. I was happy to see her try anything. Now we both use the O Loop, though I use it more during masturbation than sex because I like to focus on her process and help her."

—Megan, 31

"Her O Loop took the pressure off me to make it happen for her. I was raised by a feminist mother. That popular seventies expression 'I am responsible for my own orgasm!' was in my consciousness. Then I married a woman who couldn't come and looked at me with that 'How come?' look on her face. The O Loop is great."

—Stephen, 35

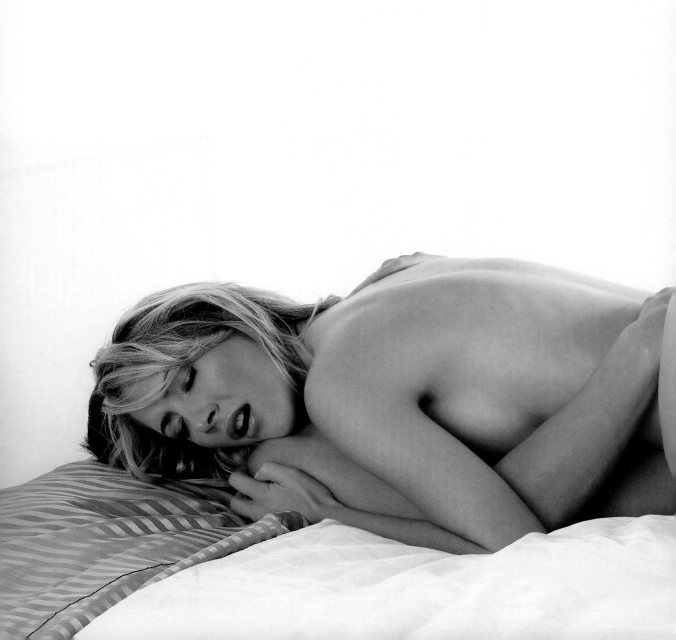

Part 3

Reaching Orgasm Every Time

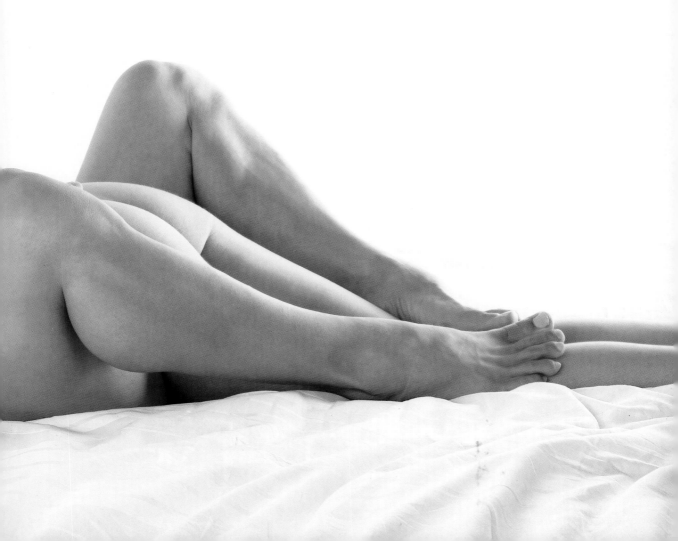

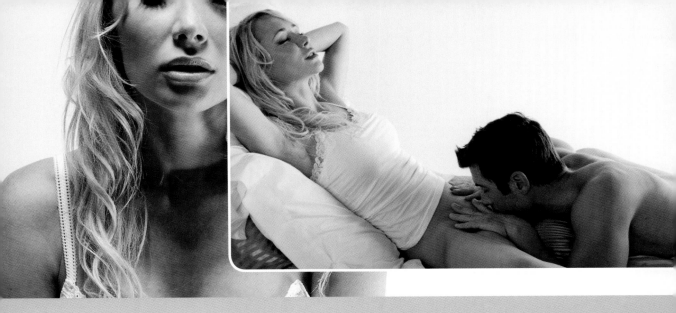

Step 4

Integrate the O Loop with Oral Play

"Many women feel that sex will go on until their partner 'gives' them an orgasm. Sometimes women fake an orgasm to end the sex and make the man feel good at the same time."

—Dr. Ruth Westheimer, therapist and author

"LADIES FIRST" doesn't mean the same thing today as it did when men held doors for women, ordered for them in restaurants, and handed them into the lifeboats first. These days, it means he gives her the first orgasm via cunnilingus. Then he takes his release during intercourse.

Many men feel that they must "give" a woman an orgasm via cunnilingus before they have their own. In spite of this gallant behavior, men are maligned as self-centered lovers just because women don't reach orgasm during intercourse alone and men do. The truth is that most men want their partners to have an orgasm as much as they want to experience their own pleasure. A man measures his ability as a lover in his partner's orgasm. Maybe he (and she) would be happier if her orgasms came more often during intercourse—but he is not to blame for this cultural bias that is based on machismo myth and machisma romance, not biology. It's cultural myth that we all subscribe to; women and men believe that she should come during intercourse alone. According to his myth, his penis should be enough. Her myth also says his penis should be enough— if it's true love. We have all played a part in creating and validating this intercourse-centric belief system. (Remember, I invented the Orgasm Loop in response to that question women never stop asking: How can I come during intercourse?)

In fact, couples may not acknowledge this to one another, but:

- She doesn't expect to have a second orgasm during intercourse and might fake the one he thinks she's having.
- He is only sure she's had an orgasm if he's performing oral sex, and he suspects she's faking the second one anyway.

Consequently, cunnilingus is the de facto essential sex technique in the modern sexual relationship—heterosexual as well as lesbian. Too bad so much weight is put on that one aspect of lovemaking. Oral sex is a pleasure for both recipient and giver, but it should not be the only reliable way a woman reaches orgasm.

See how much more you will enjoy cunnilingus when, thanks to the Orgasm Loop, you aren't counting on that most of the time.

Real Talk

"Oral sex. I rarely come any other way. I've been with my husband for ten years, five years married, but it was the same story with my previous boyfriends. Every now and then I hear some woman complain about a man who won't go down. And I think: Does she ever come with him?"

—Jane, 40

"Cunnilingus. I have been with guys who didn't do that or didn't do it well. I never came. I just faked. They seemed okay with that. I learned to separate sex—what I did with the man—from orgasm—what I got on my own when I masturbated."

—Christie, 36

"Oral and manual. It's not about the dick when you're talking about coming. I love the dick anyway. My new favorite way to come is humping my guy's leg while I give him head."

—Jasmine, 27

What Is Your Lover's Cunnilingus Style?

Some men love to perform cunnilingus and delight in the sensations of a woman's vagina. Others do it because it gets the job done. They just want her to come so they can move on to what they really like, intercourse.

There are men who learned everything they know about cunnilingus from porn films. They favor flashy full-tongue licks, the moves that show a lot of tongue in close-ups. And they alternate big tongue moves with pressing their faces hard against her. The nose-to-clitoris stroke is a new favorite among this group.

And there are men who have learned from their lovers. They are more likely to use the tips of their tongues to great advantage. Their touch is more delicate, quick, and sure. They pay close attention to their partner's responses and adjust the speed and angle of tongue play to accommodate.

His style might affect how easily you can integrate the O Loop into cunnilingus. The best way to get what you want from him without losing your arousal or energy-moving focus is to get into the right position. Here are the basic cunnilingus positions and how they work with his style and your O Loop.

What the Research Says

CAN MEN TELL THE DIFFERENCE?

In a recent 2007 study of couples reported by the Pew Research Center (Washington, D.C., U.S.), 36 percent of women said they were faking orgasms with their male partners. Only 14 percent of those men reported that their lovers were faking. These numbers were even higher in a 2006 Danish study on sexual satisfaction, in which 80 percent of Danish women said they faked orgasms, and only 17 percent of Danish men in the same study said women had faked orgasms with them.

Any woman can fake any man any time. The physical signs generally regarded as proof of orgasm—elevated pulse rate, flushed chest, rapid breathing—can also be "signs of energy put into a good fake job or just arousal that didn't lead to orgasm," according to relationship expert and psychotherapist Nan Wise. "You can't be sure a woman has had an orgasm without an MRI."

The Cunnilingus Positions

Sitting

You are sitting in bed with your back against the headboard. Or you are sitting in a chair, your legs open, knees bent, and feet on the floor. In bed, your legs are likely outstretched and open, forming a V. In either case, your lover is kneeling or lying between your legs.

Your lover is in the power position because you don't have freedom to move. He (or she) has you wedged between the backrest and his mouth. That makes this a place you don't want to be while O Looping if his approach to cunnilingus is large, forceful, and wet. (On the other hand, if he has a particularly talented tongue, this classic cunnilingus position works fine with the O Loop.)

The O Loop Adaptation: Leverage some more space for yourself by putting pillows behind your back. (They can be pulled out one at a time if you need to move back from him.) And ask him to use that tongue on your inner thighs, your belly button, and the backs of your knees. Tell him you are looking for new hot spots for him to stimulate while you O Loop.

If his aggressive approach makes you lose focus, put your feet on his shoulders and create some distance, or pull the pillows out from behind you and stretch out on the bed into the next position.

Reclining

Lying flat on your back in bed, you may elevate your head on the pillow or not. Your legs can be open wide and stretched out on the bed. Or you may have your feet flat on the bed, knees bent, legs open. He kneels or lies flat between your legs. He may hold on to your legs as he performs cunnilingus.

This is a good position for keeping him from grinding his face into you when you don't want that. You can push your legs against his hands or bring your knees together gently around the sides of his head. Most lovers will take that as a cue.

The O Loop Adaptation: Or flip to the female superior position, straddle his face, and lower your clitoris to his mouth.

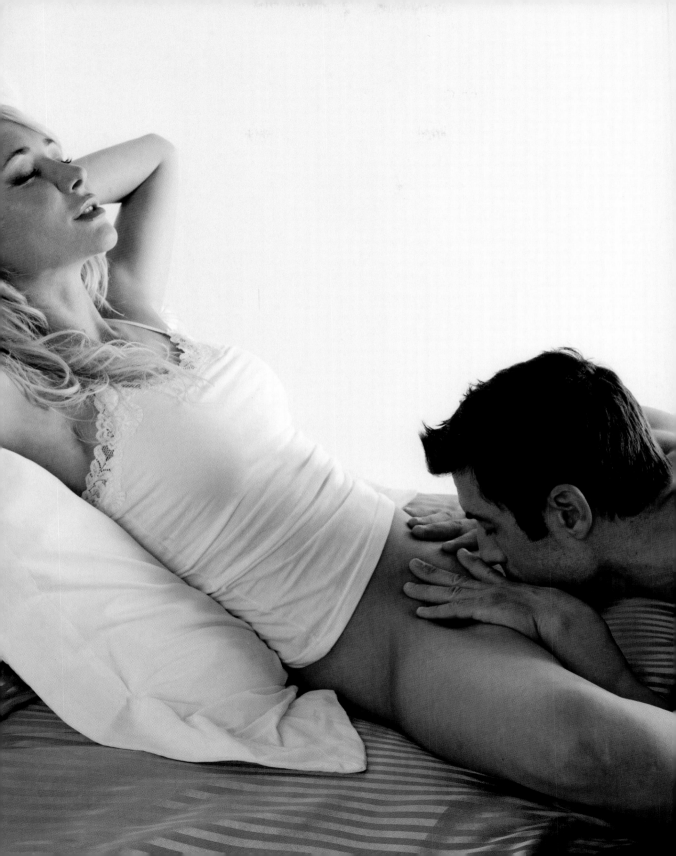

Standing

In the ultimate power position, you are standing, feet apart, while he kneels between your legs. You have more range of movement than he does. There is no pressure on your body. If you have a door frame or something else to grasp, you can also anchor yourself.

The O Loop Adaptation: Steady yourself by placing your hands on his shoulders and leaning slightly forward against him. As you fire breathe, imagine the fire coming through his mouth and into your genitals.

Rear Entry

You are on hands and knees in the same position you use for rear-entry intercourse. Your chest may be lowered onto the bed or not. He kneels behind you and comes at your clitoris from this different angle, or he lies beneath you with his head centered under your genitals.

The O Loop Adaptation: If he is behind you, push back and forth against him, thrusting gently into his mouth, so that he feels your PC flexing. He will likely get into your rhythm. When he's beneath you, ride his mouth. Again, he will pick up your rhythm. Imagine that circle of fire shooting out the tip of his tongue and into your body.

Tired Tongue?

The Tongue is a vibe that looks and performs like a real tongue. And it rotates! Use it alone to simulate cunnilingus, or have your partner make it his "assistant."

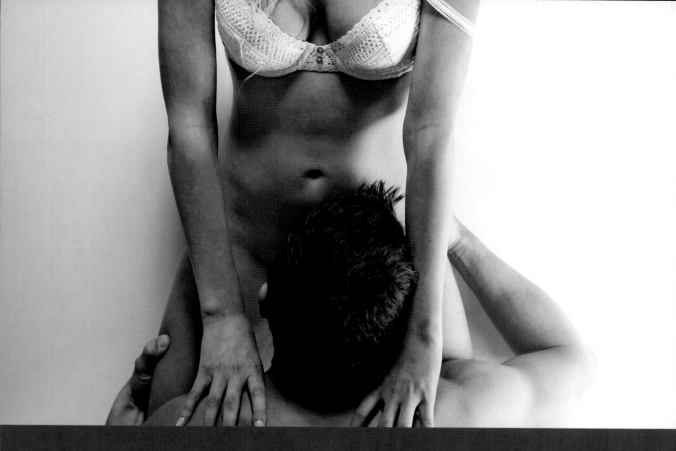

CUNNILINGUS TECHNIQUES

You can show (or read) this to your lover, or not.

Gently part her labia. Holding her lips open, lift the clitoral hood. If her clitoris is well back inside the hood—an "innie"—gently run your fingers along the side of the hood to expose the clitoris. (You might have to keep one hand in this position.)

Lick the delicate tissue along the sides and above and below her clitoris in long, broad, gentle strokes of the tongue.

Put your lips around the sides of her clitoris. Hold them in a pursed position as you gently suck. Alternate the sucking with licking of the surrounding tissue.

Cover the clitoral shaft area with your mouth. Suck gently around the sides of her clitoris. Stimulate her labia with your hand, stroke her inner thighs, or tease her nipples, or alternate oral play with manual stimulation.

Real Talk

"I asked my boyfriend of six months to use a light touch so I
could keep my focus. Really, I have wanted to tell him to lighten
up for some time but didn't know how. He took the instruction
beautifully! And I didn't have any problems O Looping. Everything
seemed to flow together. He was matching his tongue strokes to
my PC flexing and breathing."

—Carmen, 28

"At a certain point, I lose track of O Looping, but it doesn't matter.
I am about to come at that point anyway."

—Keisha, 23

"I wasn't completely comfortable with receiving oral sex before
I started O Looping. My ex-husband didn't go there. I am into
my own arousal and energy moving now, so I don't have those
nagging little worries about how I smell and taste to him. It all
worked out fine."

—Nadia, 49

Can You O Loop and Perform Fellatio at the Same Time?

Yes, you can, as long as you are comfortable using the O Loop and also confident of your fellatio skills. Not so sure about that oral technique? Use the directions below and practice before adding the O Loop.

But why try to combine the O Loop and fellatio? If you lose your arousal and energy focus while you're performing fellatio, you may have trouble getting back into the O Loop, particularly if he is ready to move to intercourse now. Keeping your arousal high isn't the only reason for combining the two. Especially if you really enjoy performing fellatio, you might experience that rare event, a fellatio orgasm.

Some women do reach orgasm this way. And I'm not talking about the women who add clitoral stimulation by rubbing their genitals against his body or masturbating as they fellate him. Maybe 10 percent of women can come while performing fellatio simply by flexing their PC muscles in time with their mouth movements. Add fire breathing, arousal focus, and energy moving, and surely the odds go way up.

The Basic Black Dress of Blow Jobs

Kiss and lick his inner thighs while pulling down ever so slightly on his scrotum. With your finger pads, scratch his testicles. Put his balls carefully into your mouth one at a time. Roll them around. Then, again, ever so gently, pull them down with your mouth. While you're attending to his balls, run your fingers lovingly up and down the shaft of his penis.

Get into a comfortable position, kneeling at his side on the bed or at a right angle to his body or kneeling between his legs. Or you can bring him down to the edge of the bed and kneel on the floor. Wet your lips and make sure they cover your teeth. Run your tongue around the head of his penis to moisten it.

Hold the base of his penis firmly in one hand. With the other hand, you can form a circle with your thumb and forefinger, what sex expert Lou Paget calls "the "ring and the seal," to elongate your mouth and prevent him from going in farther than you would like. Use that hand in a twisting motion as you fellate him. Or, if his erection is not firm, you can use both hands (wrapped around the shaft) in an upward twist stroke.

Circle the head with your tongue in a swirling motion, and then work your tongue in long strokes up and down his shaft. Now, back to the head.

SWALLOWING

If you don't stop the blow job before he comes, you have two options: swallow or let his semen dribble out of your mouth.

Swallowing is not really difficult, and he will love you for it. A man feels totally accepted and loved by a woman who swallows his semen.

Position yourself so that his ejaculate will shoot straight down your throat. An easy way of doing this is to lie on your back with your head off the bed. Your mouth and throat will form a smooth line. Have him straddle your face for the elegant finish to the perfect blow job.

Real Talk

DID YOU COME PERFORMING FELLATIO WITH THE O LOOP?

"No, but I kept my arousal going. Our routine had always been: I get the first oral orgasm, we have intercourse for a while, and I finish him off orally. He was really surprised when I stopped fellating him, climbed on top—and had a second orgasm."

—Elaine, 45

"Yes! If I'm into a man, I'm really into sucking him. I am a phallocentric woman. Using the O Loop, I have orgasms giving him head. I feel the flexing and breathing in my throat and I feel his cock pulsating inside my mouth. It's incredible. We both love this."

—Kim, 33

Follow the ridge of the corona (the ridge separating the head from the shaft) with your tongue while working the shaft with your hands, the penis sandwiched between them.

With your tongue, strum the frenulum (the loose section of skin on the underside of the penis, where the head meets the shaft). Lick the raphe, the visible line along the center of the scrotum.

Make eye contact with him from time to time.

Do at least ten to twenty seconds of this showy move: repeatedly pull his penis into your mouth, then push it out, using suction while keeping the tongue in motion.

Go back to the head. Swirl your tongue around it. Suck the head. Swirl. Suck. Repeat. Repeat.

Follow his lead if he pulls back from stimulation. He's telling you that he's going to reach orgasm if you don't stop.

69: Hot—or Not?

The mutual oral sex position "69" typically looks hotter than it feels. Most people get a little lazy in their technique when they are highly aroused by the oral attention they're receiving at the other end of the body curve. A "69" typically devolves into "do me/then I do you," with the passive (recipient) partner stimulating the other's genitals manually, not orally.

It's not a good position if you're an O Loop beginner, because maintaining the balance of giving and receiving pleasure takes away from your focus. If "69" is something your partner enjoys, do it after you have reached orgasm with the O Loop and want to shift into sex play that is more about him than you.

Rekindling the Joy of Oral

The Orgasm Loop can add another dimension to oral sex, both the giving and the receiving of it. If you and your partner have fallen into the habit of you receiving your orgasm via cunnilingus, the O Loop makes the experience richer. And you don't have to regard fellatio as something you do just for him now. With the Loop, you can come, too.

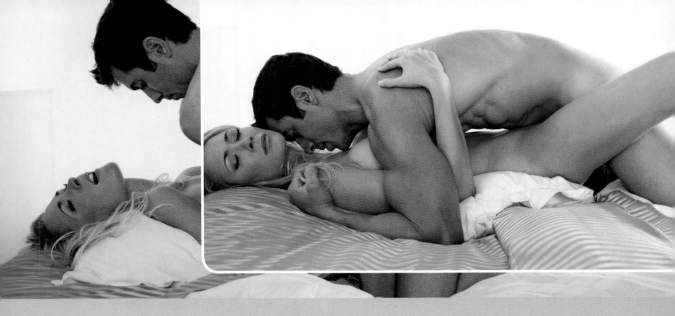

Step 5

The Big O—Use the O Loop During Intercourse

> " Clearly orgasm represents a lot more than the few moments of neuropsychological release by which it's clinically defined . . . orgasm both gratifies and confounds us in ways that transcend our biology."
>
> —Nina Hartley, author of *Nina Hartley's Guide to Total Sex*

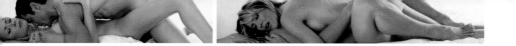

FOR MANY WOMEN, this is the gold chapter, the one that answers the question: How can I have an orgasm during intercourse?

The quick answer is: Use your hand. But women who ask the question really mean: how can I have a no-hands orgasm during intercourse? Even women who understand that unassisted intercourse orgasms aren't naturally favored by female anatomy and physiology still want it to happen.

Now that using the Orgasm Loop is like swimming or riding a bike—skills you never forget how to use—you can have the no-hands intercourse orgasm.

How to Use the Orgasm Loop During Intercourse

There are six basic intercourse positions, as well as numerous variations on each one. Any position can work with the O Loop. You may initially want to make minor adaptations to positions for two reasons:

- It may be easier for you to sustain your breathing and flexing rhythms in some positions than others because you have more control over the speed and depth of his thrusting.
- You may opt for positions where you don't face each other; those are less "intimate" and allow you to maintain your focus. (After using the O Loop during intercourse a few times, you probably won't need to protect your focus.)

Real Talk

"Having an orgasm during intercourse is a deeply emotionally
satisfying experience. On the one hand, I know how bodies work
and this is a shallow and silly aspiration—an adult woman's
sexual manifestation of the princess myth. On the other hand,
I want it. I love the way it feels when he comes inside me and I
want that feeling for him, too."

—Rhonda, 33

"It's only important to me if I am in a relationship. Now I am
seeing someone, but it's not serious, it's just sex. I am working
my O Loop without telling him and reaching orgasm during
intercourse, which thrills him, but it's all just practice. I would
masturbate myself to orgasm with this guy if that's what I
needed to do."

—Laura, 29

"I think every woman, if she's honest with herself, wants to come
during intercourse alone. She wants to be that sexy, responsive
woman who is swept away to ecstasy on the strength of his
thrusting. Using your hand makes it all so mechanical. Where is
the magic? We need more magic in our sex lives."

—Katie, 52

The Intercourse Positions

Missionary Position

Women usually rate this position more favorably than men do. (Over the past decade, numerous women's and men's magazines from *Redbook* to *Playboy* have run surveys that say she likes rear entry and missionary, while he favors rear entry and female superior.) In the basic missionary position, she lies on her back with her legs slightly parted, and he lies on top of her, supporting himself at least partially with his hands.

Some variations that favor female orgasm:

- Place a pillow(s) beneath the small of your back to change the angle of penetration to one of greater depth.
- Lie on your back with your legs up as straight and high as they will comfortably go. He kneels in front of you. This tightens your vagina, providing greater friction for both of you—and it leaves your hands free to play with your clitoris.
- Lie on your back and put your legs over his shoulders.
- Lift one leg up and put it over his shoulder or around his back.
- Put your feet on his chest or shoulders, again to change the angle of penetration and control the thrust.
- Wrap your legs around his waist or his neck for the same reasons.
- Sit on the edge of the bed. He either holds your legs or you wrap them around him as he enters you from a standing position.

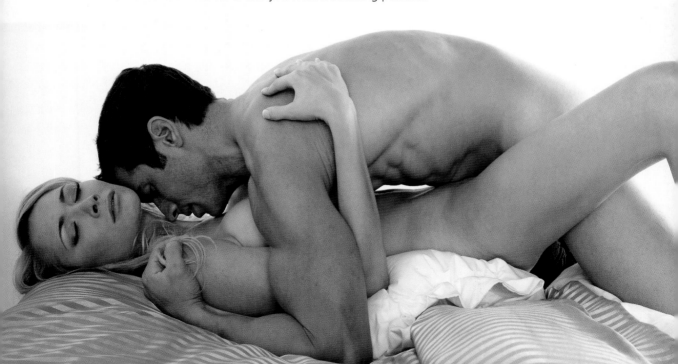

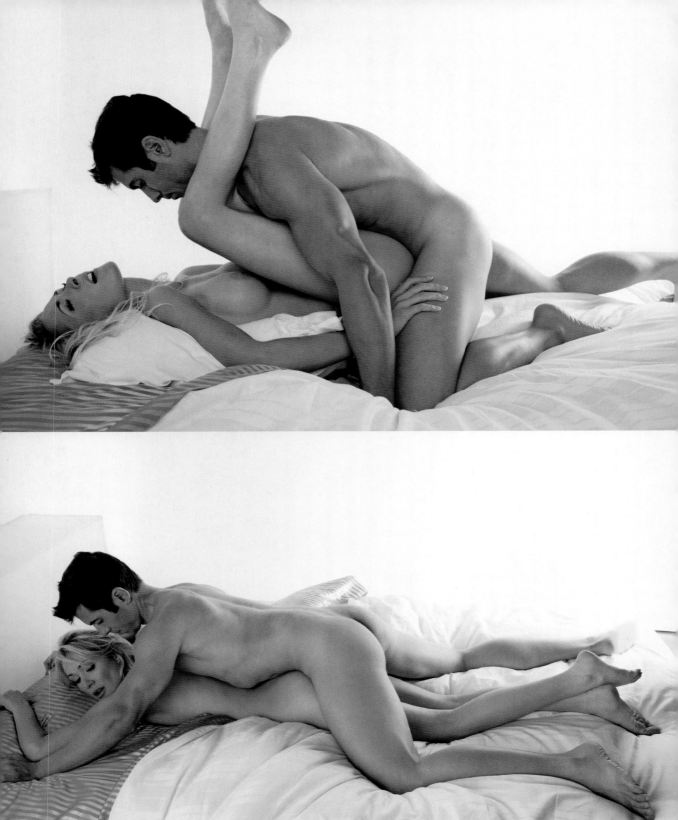

The O Loop Adaptation (pictured):

1. **Put a pillow under your shoulders so that you can throw your head back and close your eyes.** (Big plus: This really looks hot.) Choose one of the variations where you put one or both legs over his shoulders or your feet against his chest or shoulders. You have reduced the eye contact factor (intimacy) and put yourself in better control of the thrusting.

2. **Flip it.** He's still on top, but you're not facing him. Lie on your stomach, legs straight out and spread only slightly. He lies over you, supporting his weight on his elbows. Position his legs on either side of you. As he enters you, close your legs and cross them at the ankles. Crossing your ankles and holding your legs together enables you to feel the entire length of his penis inside you. As he's thrusting, he's in a great position to kiss your neck, nibble your ears, and reach under to play with your clitoris.

   Again, you have eliminated the eye contact associated with this classic position and reduced the speed and depth of thrusting.

Side-by-Side Position

Often a favorite position for the weary couple—or the semi-erect man—side by side is sometimes called "spooning" and even "stuffing and spooning." In the basic version of the position, he faces her back. Her buttocks are angled against him as he puts one leg between hers. Or she can lie half on her back, half on her side, drawing up the leg upon which she is lying. He faces her.

Some variations that favor female orgasm:

- Add manual stimulation.
- Add a vibrator. This is a great position for vibe play (or manual stimulation) because hands are free.

The O Loop Adaptation: Use the basic variation where he faces your back. Move slightly higher than you normally would in this position, and use his leg between yours as leverage so that you are controlling the thrusting.

Rear-Entry Position

A favorite position of everyone from the ancient Chinese to the modern Western couple, rear entry is also known by its nickname, "doggy style." This position facilitates deep penetration, G-spot stimulation, and hard thrusting; it also puts her clitoris in a good place for manual stimulation. A nice bonus: her ass looks its best here, with the little wrinkles and pockets fairly well ironed out. (Who doesn't love that?) In the basic position, the woman is on all fours, with the man kneeling behind her.

Some variations that favor female orgasm:

- Lower your upper body so that your chest touches the bed. This elongates your vaginal barrel, making a "tighter" fit for his penis.
- Try rear entry lying down, with you on your stomach. Clench your thighs together after he enters you and lift one leg for deeper penetration.

The O Loop Adaptation:

1. **Ask him to caress your vulva and finger your clitoris but otherwise remain relatively still while you thrust back against him.** (Most men will grab a woman's hips or ass and control the thrusting, but this isn't conducive while you're O Looping.)

2. **Stand by the bed or chair and lean forward onto it, with him standing behind you.** Either way, you have control in what is perhaps the best beginning O Loop position because there is no eye contact.

The Sitting Position

There's a lot you can do with this one because it accommodates different levels of passion and physical energy. In the basic position, he sits in a chair or on the bed with her astride him. Penetration is shallow.

Some variations that favor female orgasm:

- Lean backward as he thrusts, and he grasps your buttocks firmly.
- Add a vibrator, especially a vibrating cock ring on him or a strap-on vibe on you.
- Sit on the kitchen counter, washer or dryer, or high bar stool— whatever is the right height for him to enter you.

The O Loop Adaptation: Sit with your back to him, your feet on the floor. Again, you have the control and the emotional space that freedom from eye contact affords you.

The Standing Position

Having intercourse while standing satisfies that occasional need for dramatic, urgent lovemaking. It's also a great way to have a quickie. Why not test the Orgasm Loop in a quickie situation? In the basic version of the position, he squats slightly while she lowers herself onto him. She wraps one leg around his waist and he holds her buttocks.

Some variations that favor female orgasm:

- Change the depth and angle of penetration by doing it on the stairs, with you one step above him.
- Stand in front of him, facing in the opposite direction, and bend slightly forward to increase G-spot stimulation.

The O Loop Adaptation: Use the stairs. Or stand on some secure surface that elevates you above him as far as comfortably possible. Wrap one leg around him. Throw your head back, which will encourage him to ravish your neck and breasts. You'll increase the drama quotient and maintain emotional privacy and control.

Real Talk

IS THAT INTERCOURSE ORGASM AS GOOD AS YOU THOUGHT IT WOULD BE?

"Yes! I feel closer and more connected to my partner now because I can come during intercourse. It shouldn't make a big difference, but it does."

—Karen, 37

"It's emotionally satisfying. I have stronger orgasms masturbating, especially with a vibe, and receiving oral sex. But there is that emotional satisfaction you feel when you come during intercourse. He feels it, too."

—DeeDee, 22

The Anal Intercourse O Loop

Heterosexual anal sex was a taboo subject until very recently. Now young men *expect* this sex act early in the dating relationship. (That doesn't mean they are, or should, be getting it from young women they hardly know.) Their older brothers and fathers may have wanted anal sex but didn't expect to receive it. These young men feel as entitled to anal sex as the older generations did to oral sex.

Some women occasionally "offer up the ass" as a special gift for husbands or lovers. Other women enjoy the practice. And it's something every woman should probably try (within a committed, monogamous relationship) at least once. The receiver of anal intercourse is in a very submissive position. That can be a powerful, exciting, and intensely intimate experience.

Use the Orgasm Loop in other intercourse positions before you try it this way. If you like anal sex, you'll like it better with the O Loop.

What the Research Says

ANAL SEX: WHO'S DOING IT?

Now this is interesting: back in the '40s and '50s, when Alfred Kinsey was collecting his data on sexual behavior, 9 percent of men and 28 percent of women reported heterosexual anal intercourse. Why so many women? Virginity was a bride's prized asset. Anal intercourse preserved her hymen. Why so few men? Surely they lied out of fear of being thought "homosexual."

In 1974, *Playboy* magazine surveyed 2,000 readers and found that, depending on the age of the respondent, 14 to 25 percent of men had participated in heterosexual anal sex, with men over forty reporting higher numbers than men in their twenties. (Finally admitting what they were doing to preserve a girlfriend's virginity in the '50s?)

More recent studies, including the 2002 National Survey of Family Growth (Department of Health and Human Services, Washington, D.C., U.S) report that about a third of both men and women have engaged in the activity at least once.

Anal Intercourse Positions

Rear Entry

While most intercourse positions can be adapted to anal sex, rear entry is probably the position most commonly used. There are two obvious reasons for that. Her anus is more accessible, and the submissive nature of the act is underscored by the position. Additionally, the classic pose allows her to push against his penis, which both aids entry and gives her some control over the speed and depth of thrusting.

The O Loop Adaptation: It's time for some eye contact now. You are comfortable using the O Loop during intercourse, so you don't need the private space. And it's good for him to see your face and read in it any discomfort you may be feeling. Lie on your back, with your knees on your chest. He still has easy access. You have greater control and are in a more comfortable position that is easier to maintain through the slower thrusting.

YOGA SEXERCISES FOR TWO

The anus and surrounding tissues are highly sensitive to erotic touch. These two exercises contract the anus to build heightened sensitivity in the area.

The Horse Gesture

Sit in a cross-legged yoga position. Inhale deeply and hold the breath briefly. As you exhale slowly, contract the sphincter muscles, pulling the anus up and in. Repeat. Do a set of ten a day the first week. Build to twenty a day. Do one set a day for a month, then do two or three sets a week.

The Root Lock

This is a more advanced version of the horse gesture. Again, sit in the yoga position. Or lie on your back with your knees bent, if that is more comfortable for you. About halfway through a deep breath, contract your sphincter muscles. Expand the breath and the contraction from the anus through the PC, into the genitals. Men will feel a pull in the testicles and women a quiver in the labia. Start with ten a day and work up to twenty. Do one set a day for a month, then do two or three sets a week.

A GUIDE TO SAFE ANAL PENETRATION

Share this tip with your lover—either a man or a woman wearing a strap-on. (And read it yourself if you will be wearing the strap-on, too.)

Always use a specially designed anal condom and PLENTY of a lubricant like Astroglide. (The anus, unlike the vagina, is not self-lubricating.) The condom is essential to keep bacteria out of your urethra. Using a finger protected by a disposable "finger cot," insert copious amounts of lube into her anus.

Start very slowly.

As you press the head of your penis against her anus, encourage her to relax the sphincter muscles in her rectum.

Don't force your penis inside her. Ask her to bear down on the head of your penis until you are past the sphincter muscles.

Following her lead, thrust slowly and carefully. Let her control the depth of penetration and the speed of thrusting.

While you are thrusting, either you or she should be stimulating her clitoris. With any luck, she will reach orgasm.

Afterward, don't insert your penis into her vagina until you have removed the condom and thoroughly washed your penis and hands. You both risk contracting a urinary tract infection if the cleanliness rules are not scrupulously followed.

Take It All in Stride

There is a lot of material to absorb in this chapter, but you don't have to master it all immediately. Your goal is simply to make orgasm happen more reliably during intercourse. Take your time with the techniques and exercises. When you are comfortable with one, move on to the next. No pressure!

Real Talk

DO YOU ENJOY ANAL INTERCOURSE?

"No, but I do it occasionally. I consider it a gift to my husband. Using the O Loop made anal intercourse a better experience for me. I was focused on breathing and flexing and didn't tense up when he entered me. So it didn't hurt as much as it usually does."

—Sara, 38

"Yes, sometimes. I haven't done it with every man in my life. When I am really into a man, I like to be submissive sometimes, just as I like to be dominant sometimes, too. It's extreme sex. It hurts, but it hurts good. I reach orgasm this way with the O Loop."

—Ella, 39

"I never wanted to do it, but I got really hot once I was into it. Using the O Loop helped take the nervous edge off getting started. I was so hot—and I came! My boyfriend would love anal intercourse once a week, but it takes too much preparation and is too intense an experience."

—Annie, 30

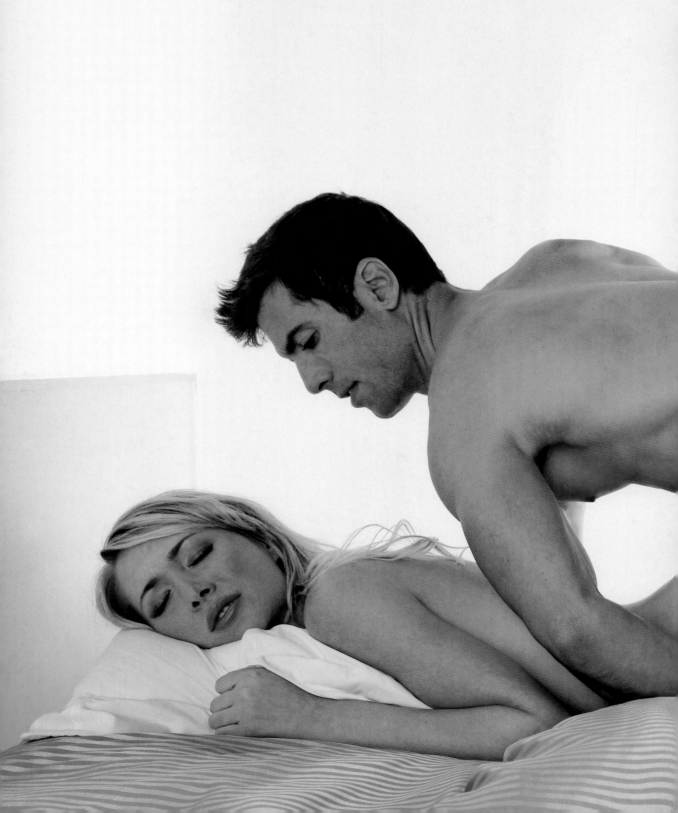

Part 4

Advanced O Looping

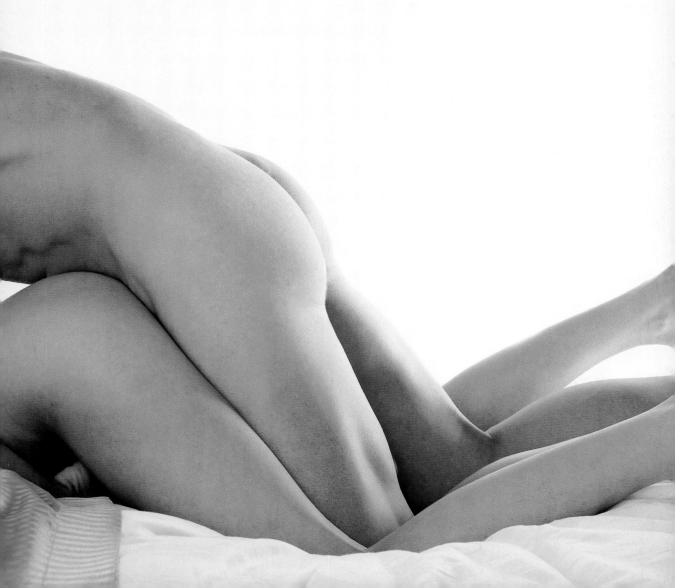

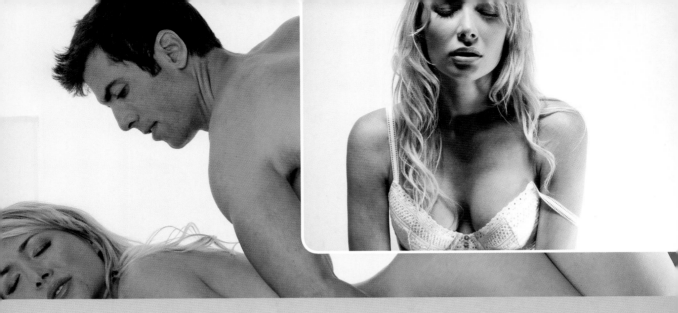

Chapter 3

The Simultaneous O Loop Orgasm

"Only women fake a simultaneous orgasm—because men believe it really happened. Women are smarter than that. Subconsciously we know women wouldn't believe that fake."

—Bob Berkowitz, Ph.D., broadcast journalist and author of *What Men Won't Tell You But Women Need to Know*

THE SIMULTANEOUS ORGASM is certainly not the norm. Most couples take turns. Yet it is a cultural ideal. It's possible that more women have faked simultaneous orgasm than have ever achieved it. Women fake an orgasm as he is ejaculating because they know he can be easily fooled at that particular moment. And the faked simultaneous O neatly ends the sex, one of the reasons women give for faking.

Why is this particular double orgasm so desirable anyway?

The image of an entwined couple writhing in ecstasy together taunts us everywhere—in novels, mainstream movies, and porn flicks. Historically, both men and women believed that his pleasure triggered hers. Some doctors in the nineteenth century actually told women that their joy at the flow of his ejaculate inside their vagina would give them an orgasm. (And then they prescribed masturbation to relieve her hysteria.) Even Kinsey said it was the "most a couple can achieve in an intimate relationship." We know that's not true, yet still we dream.

Logic aside, reaching orgasm together can make the intimate connection between two lovers feel more intense. Better, it's a thrill almost exclusive to couples, not casual lovers. The keys to simultaneous orgasm are communication and timing, and couples in long-term relationships are more familiar with each other's bodies and sexual responses than strangers are.

We are all longing for something most likely to be experienced by a couple—that couple with two jobs, kids, a mortgage, and no time or energy for sex.

Solving the Seeming Contradiction

Now here is where things really get interesting, the place where we get to the heart of the matter regarding that seeming contradiction mentioned at the beginning of this book. Why do so many reports claim women want intimacy more than orgasm, but women themselves are still asking all the time how they can have orgasms during sex?

Couples in serious, committed relationships may have the best chance of experiencing simultaneous orgasm, but as any loving couple knows, simultaneous orgasm does not always happen. And it's not always easy, especially when couples are exhausted and worn out from all of their daily responsibilities. But when simultaneous orgasm does happen, it is a very powerful physical and emotional manifestation of a couple's bond and the connection they share. That is the gold standard that everyone ultimately wants.

What women really want is both great sex and intimacy at the same time—more specifically, great sex that leads to orgasm because of the closeness and the intimacy they have with their partner. The truth is, this isn't an either/or proposition. Yes, women can have both—orgasms and intimacy. But let's be honest, we really don't want (and can't truly have) the intimacy without the orgasms. Orgasm leads to intimacy; sexual frustration does not.

So for all of you worn-out couples who are busy working and chasing the kids: how can you get to that place of great sex and simultaneous orgasm? The Orgasm Loop can help you get closer by helping her focus on her arousal. Read on in this chapter and see how.

How to Adapt Simultaneous Orgasm Techniques to the O Loop

There are three techniques for achieving simultaneous orgasm. You can use the Orgasm Loop with any or all of them, and thus increase the odds of making it happen.

Stretch Out Foreplay for Two

The method: Kiss, caress, fondle, stroke, and arouse one another via oral sex, but no orgasm allowed. Hold off on intercourse until you are both at the "high fever" state of arousal. The physical signs: panting, sweating, flushed chest, that glazed look in the eyes.

Don't move to intercourse until you get those signals. Then move together in a state of close communication with eyes open and hands on back, buttocks, or thighs ready to indicate "faster" or "slower." If one of you is closer to orgasm than the other, that partner stops moving and signals. Use a sexy code phrase like "too hot" or a touch like gently placing your hands on the other's hips and pushing your bodies slightly away from one another. Still connected though not moving, the partner on the verge kisses, caresses, and strokes the other.

The partner who signals for a brief halt in stimulation gets the slow-down he or she needs while continuing to give the erotic attention the other needs to keep his or her arousal building. The less aroused partner continues to receive the kissing, stroking, and caressing he or she needs to catch up. Look into one another's eyes now if you are comfortable doing that because eye contact during intercourse will help you gauge how close you each are to release, helping you time the movements. The more dilated those pupils are, the closer you each are to orgasm. Once you are both in the same place, move together again to simultaneous orgasms.

The O Loop Adaptation: Using the O Loop, you will reach the state of high arousal more quickly than you have in the past. Ask your partner to pay close attention to your arousal and keep pace with you. When you are near orgasm, take charge. In the female superior position, you control the angle and depth of thrusting. Because your PC muscle is well developed and strong, you can bring him along to orgasm by contracting and releasing rapidly as you come.

Finish Oral Foreplay with a Fancy "69"

The method: He's hot; you're not exactly. When you start lovemaking with this arousal imbalance, he typically performs cunnilingus until you have the first orgasm. Then he takes his. This time he stops before you come so you forego the "ladies first" prerogative. When he has stimulated you to the verge of orgasm, pull back by gently taking his face in your hands and moving your hips back at the same time. As soon as you send him this physical signal, he understands that you are near orgasm. He, on the other hand, might need a little extra stimulation to catch up. Ask him whether he wants oral or manual pleasuring, and give him enough to bring him up to your speed. Get into the "69" position.

The O Loop Adaptation: You start in the "69" position, but he initially gives you more oral attention than you give him. You fellate him enough to maintain his erection until you are on the verge of orgasm. Then you match his pace.

The Adapted C.A.T. Position

The method: The Coital Alignment Technique—an adaptation of the missionary position that puts his full weight on her—has been touted as the no-fail simultaneous orgasm position. (The caveat: it's very uncomfortable for a woman if her husband is bigger than she is.) Lie on your back. With his pelvis higher than yours, he enters you, putting his full weight on your body. (If he's a lot taller, his chin will be resting on top of your head because he has to move his pelvis as high as it will go while sustaining the intercourse connection.) Wrap your legs around his thighs, resting your ankles on his calves. Move only your pelvises in a steady rhythm, without speeding up or slowing down, until you reach orgasm together.

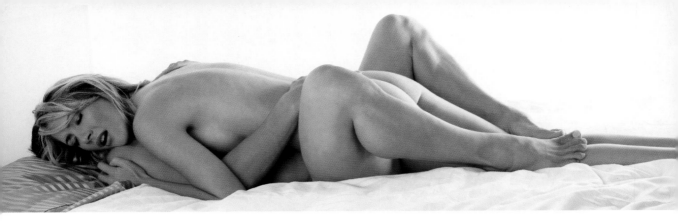

The direct, continuous stimulation this position provides your clitoris enables you need to reach orgasm during intercourse alone. Plus, the constraints the position places on his movement naturally slow him down, which makes you more likely to be in sync. He can't move too vigorously, and at the same time he gives you that steady stimulation right on target.

The O Loop Adaptation: Using the O Loop, you don't need as much time in the C.A.T. position, which was designed for slowly bringing a woman to orgasm via friction against her clitoris. Bring him down to eye contact level. Lock pelvises and wrap your legs around his thighs while he supports most of his weight on his arms.

Another way of opening up the C.A.T. is by lifting his weight off you. He grasps the headboard, using that to support his weight, and leverages his movements against you.

Or you can reverse the C.A.T., with you on top, lying flat against him, pelvises locked, his legs wrapped around your body.

In any variation, speed up or slow down that "steady rhythm" to suit your own timing needs. Let your breathing and flexing set the pace.

Try, Try Again

Whether you are in a long-term relationship or a new one, there are times you want to feel closer. The Orgasm Loop can help you make that happen. But don't feel like a failure if you don't reach orgasm simultaneously. Just remember that old cliché: practice makes perfect!

Real Talk

WHAT IS YOUR SIMULTANEOUS ORGASM SECRET?

"As a joke, we used our nightstand clock to time how long it took for each of us to move from arousal to orgasm. But we realized that we could change the dynamic of intercourse by extending the time he spent giving me foreplay, as long as I barely reciprocated. That led us to see which kissing and caressing strokes were more effective than others. We got the payoff in a simultaneous orgasm. When I started using the O Loop, I had the power to make it happen because I could control my arousal."

—Denise, 32

"We did fall into that typical lovemaking pattern of 'she comes first.' It was so easy! To come at the same time, we agreed on a signal for pulling back from oral stimulation when I was 'close.' We needed a clear signal that wasn't like anything I typically did. So I tweaked his nipple. That worked. "

—Carolyn, 29

"We tried the C.A.T. without adaptation and both hated it. I was smothered and he felt constrained. But keeping our pelvises locked as we moved rhythmically together did work for us, both when he supported himself on his arms and when I was on top. The secret is in holding that pelvis connection really tight and keeping the movements in sync with my fire breathing and PC flexing."

—Cassie, 28

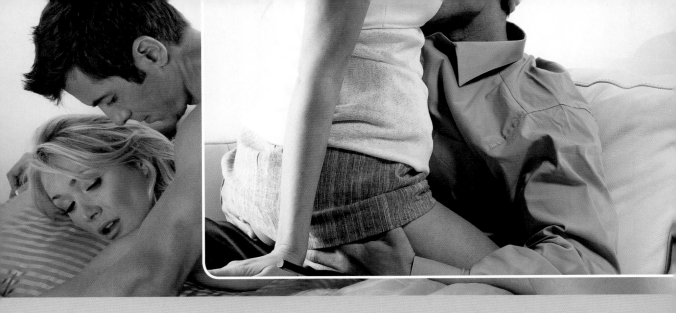

Chapter 4

The Ultimate Quickie

"Nothing takes a couple out of their sexual rut like a quickie. Brief sexual encounters are good even if they don't end in orgasm. They spark libido."

—Barbara Keesling, Ph.D., therapist and author of *The Good Girl's Guide to Bad Girl Sex*

THE FORMERLY MALIGNED intercourse quickie is getting new respect these days. Once couples assumed that a quickie was something she occasionally did "just for him," because she couldn't possibly come fast enough to make it work for her. And wasn't a quickie his idea because he was the one in a hurry? According to conventional wisdom, she wanted extended lovemaking sessions. That was your mother's (or your grandmother's) quickie. You are just as time-pressured, if not more so, than your man. And you can make this position work for you as well as him.

According to Dr. Joel Block, author of *The Art of the Quickie*, men and women naturally have an eleven-minute arousal difference. Making a quickie work is simply a matter of cutting that differential down. The Orgasm Loop can help you do that.

How to Adapt the O Loop to Quickie Techniques

Several techniques make the quickie more female-orgasm friendly. These include:

- Start on "hot." Sometimes, a quickie calls for a bit of premeditation or advance planning, as in "I'll be there in ten minutes" or "Meet me in the bathroom after you put the baby down." Because nothing gets you there as quickly as focused self-pleasuring, masturbate (not to orgasm) alone in the bathroom or bedroom before the quickie event. That way, you can bring yourself to his arousal level in a few minutes.

- Masturbate yourself during intercourse.

- Adjust any position to facilitate your hot-spot connection (see below for more information). Step up onto a little stool in the standing position, put pillows behind your back or under your ass, and make whatever physical adjustments are necessary to get that hot connection immediately.

- Fantasize. Occasionally, everyone fantasizes during intercourse. If you have a "favorite fantasy" that arouses you highly, use it now.

- Prepare your body. Sometimes you may be the one making the booty call, knowing he will walk in the door ready to go. Use a lube like Liquid Silk or the new KY vaginal moisturizer (in applicators like tampons) that you can put in a little ahead of time. If you know you only have ten or fifteen minutes for your quickie, it's wise to spend a minute or two on prep.

The O Loop Adaptation:

1. **Inserting a vaginal moisturizer in advance is a good idea.**
   (Carry a single-use applicator in your handbag so you will always be prepared for spontaneous sex. Also see the hot-spot information below.) As you sometimes do with the intercourse O Loop, jump-start your arousal with a small vibe like the Pocket Rocket or a finger or lipstick vibe. Keep that vibe in your pocket or on your finger in case you need it during the quickie. (A small vibe is another useful handbag accessory.)

2. **In place of your favorite fantasy, focus on your arousal image.**
   Then use the O Loop as you usually do during intercourse, but speed up the fire breathing and PC flexing.

Hot Spots

When you have the time for luxurious masturbation or lovemaking, experiment with stimulation to your (and your lover's) "hot spots," those magical erotic places that are extremely sensitive to touch, both oral and manual. You know where most of them are, but you and your lover may not be hitting them effectively during masturbation, foreplay, oral sex, and intercourse. And you need to know how to do that during a quickie.

Her Hot Spots

The C-Spot (Her Clitoris)

The small pink organ, often compared to the penis because of its similar shape, is located at the point where the inner labia join at the top of the vaginal opening. The clitoris and the surrounding tissue, or clitoral hood, is the most sexually sensitive part of a woman's body.

The G-Spot

That small mass of rough tissue about a third of the way up the front vaginal wall was named after the German gynecologist Ernst Grafenberg, who "discovered" it in the 1940s. In fact, the authors of the Kama Sutra wrote about this area thousands of years ago. The G-spot swells when stimulated and, in some women, produces orgasm.

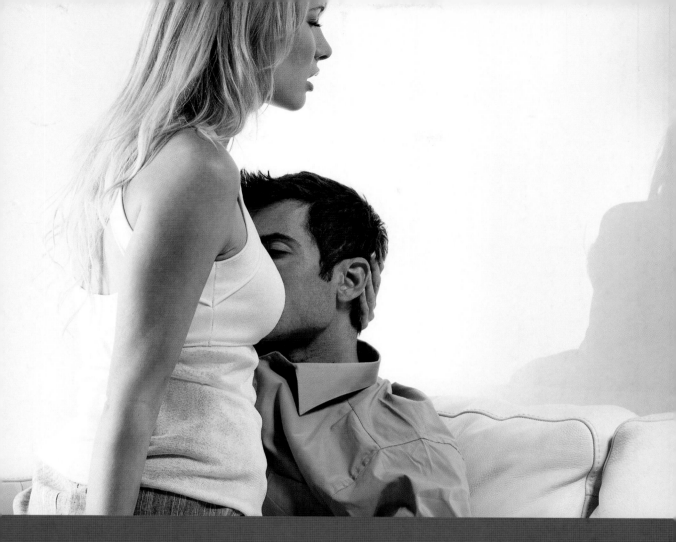

What the Research Says

HOW LONG DOES "SEX" LAST?

Statistics typically cite that from foreplay to orgasm, sex takes ten to fifteen minutes, with actual intercourse lasting two minutes. Even men think sex should last longer on average.

A 2004 *Maxim* magazine survey found that 32 percent of women said sex should last "until I orgasm" and 44 percent answered "as long as possible." Nearly 34 percent of men also said that sex should last until she has an orgasm, but only 28 percent wanted it to last as long as possible.

The AFE-Zone

The anterior fornix erotic (AFE) zone is a small patch of skin at the top of the vagina closer to the cervix than the G-spot is. Stroking the AFE Zone makes any woman lubricate immediately. Explore the front wall of your vagina with one finger. When you feel moisture forming beneath your finger, you've hit the AFE zone.

The U-Spot

We don't think of the urethra as a sexy place. But the tiny area of tissue above the opening (and right below the clitoris) is a pleasure point. This is a good spot for him to stimulate if her clitoris is too sensitive for immediate touch following orgasm.

Individual Hot Spots

Some women have very sensitive breasts or nipples. Other potential hot spots include the inner thighs, back of the knees, hollow of the throat, and back of the neck.

His Hot Spots

The H-Spot

Who doesn't know that the head of his penis is his hottest spot? Don't neglect the corona, that thick ridge of skin separating the head from the shaft. It is exquisitely sensitive to touch. Running a finger or a tongue around it can drive a man wild.

The F-Spot

The frenulum is that loose section of skin on the underside of the penis where the head meets the shaft. In most men, it is highly sensitive to touch.

The R-Area

The raphe is that visible line along the center of the scrotum, an area of the male anatomy too often overlooked during lovemaking. The skin of the scrotum is very sensitive, similar to a woman's labia.

The P-Zone

The perineum is an area an inch or so in size, between the anus and the base of the scrotum. Rich in nerve endings, the perineum is the second most important hot spot for some men—and, sadly, the hot spot many women neglect.

The G-Spot

Yes, he has one, too; it is located inside his body behind the perineum. You can reach it in two ways: indirectly, by pressing the perineum with your thumb or finger, or directly, by inserting a finger inside his anus and using the same "come hither" stroke that he uses on your G-spot.

Individual Hot Spots

Some men are very sensitive to touch on their earlobes, neck, inner thighs, temples, eyelids, nipples, and buttocks.

Real Talk

HOW LONG IS A QUICKIE?

"That depends on how much time you have for it. My guy and I have done it in a few minutes—in an elevator—and taken more than twice as long when we did it in his office after work. More than ten minutes, and it's not a quickie."

—Gailyn, 40

"Five to ten minutes. That is long enough to come if you start hot and use the O Loop."

—Andrea, 38

"As long as it takes for me to reach orgasm under optimum conditions—under ten minutes."

—Jamie, 29

QUICKIE TIPS

There are a few essential elements to a good quickie: You cannot wait to have sex, so there's no time to remove your clothes. And, the risk of discovery or interruption is present. You kiss and grab one another with urgency.

The two best quickie positions are standing and sitting, especially in a leather office chair or a chaise lounge on the patio after midnight. No drama, no quickie.

The Quickie Bonus

If you have frequent quickies, you will redefine sex. And that's a good thing.

"Sex" doesn't always have to be a period of foreplay, including oral stimulation, ending in intercourse. A quickie—or quick sex—can be oral sex for one or both in the backseat of the car parked in the garage while the kids are doing their homework. Sometimes it can be quick sex for you only, and sometimes it can be all about your lover. The time constraints of a quickie accompanied by the passionate desire for release (or just sexual contact) can inspire creativity.

You can skip the foreplay, or make it nothing but foreplay. Whatever you choose to do, frequent quickies will boost your desire level. The more sex you have, the more you will want. You don't want to treat sex like the good china—something that only gets used on special occasions!

Real Talk

"I gave a blow job to a security guard—someone I barely
knew from college—in one of the Smithsonian museums
in Washington, D.C. Before I turned a corner and saw him,
I didn't know that he was working there between semesters.
The electricity was immediate. He led me into a little storage area.
I was so excited by doing it that I went home and masturbated."

—Lauren, 24

"My husband picked me up at the office. We were alone and he
said, 'Let's live one of our fantasies.' We did it rear entry with
me bending over the desk. The next day I found my panties
in a drawer. The cleaning lady must have picked them up from
the floor and put them there."

—Catherine, 47

"I'd never been with a woman, but I had a girl crush on a woman
in my book group. We did it standing up in a pantry while the
other women argued about the social relevance of chick lit in
the living room. We rubbed against each other and kissed and
used our hands. It was so hot. We both came."

—Julia, 38

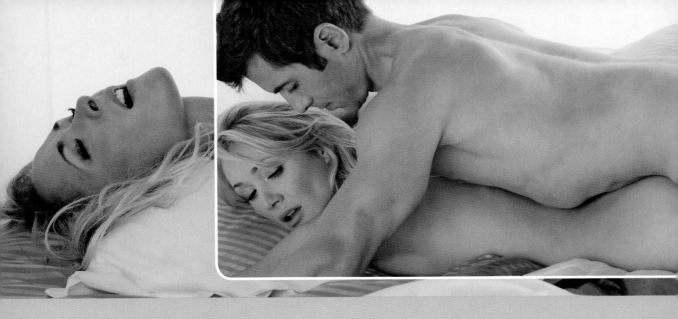

Chapter 5

Multiple O Loop Orgasms

"If you want to have multiple orgasms, you have to stay up there after the first one. Let yourself come all the way back down and you may not make the climb again until next time."

—Dr. Patti Britton, therapist, author, and president of the American Association of Sex Educators, Counselors, and Therapists (AASECT)

WOMEN WHO HAVE DIFFICULTY reaching orgasm once during lovemaking often discount multiple orgasms as the orgasm equivalent of those perfectly air-brushed bodies in the glossy magazines: unattainable models of excellence, and probably not altogether real, anyway.

Multiple orgasms are a regular occurrence for some women and definitely attainable for almost any woman. (Caveat: If you are seventy-five and you recently experienced your first orgasm—maybe not.) I don't think you should put it on the must-do list under "Kegels." But reach for multiples using the O Loop in the most playful way. This is not The Orgasm Challenge.

What Are Multiple Orgasms?

An orgasm is an intense, pleasurable response to physical, psychological, and emotional stimulation, a relaxation of sexual tension marked by a series of genital contractions and the release throughout the body of natural chemicals that create feelings of euphoria and attachment. After a single orgasm, a woman's arousal begins to subside with the last contraction. When she's having multiple orgasms, her arousal doesn't subside. It might ebb slightly. Some women report multiple orgasms as feeling like a series of waves.

There are four types of multiple orgasms:

1. **Compounded single orgasms:** Each orgasm is distinct, separated by sufficient time so that prior arousal and tension have substantially resolved between orgasms.

2. **Sequential multiples:** Orgasms are fairly close together—anywhere from two to ten minutes apart—with little interruption in sexual stimulation or level of arousal.

3. **Serial multiples:** Orgasms are separated by seconds, or up to two or three minutes, with no or barely any interruption in stimulation or diminishment of arousal.

4. **Blended multiples:** A mix of two or more of the above types. Very often women who are multiply orgasmic experience more than one type of multiple orgasms during a lovemaking session.

And for women who experience G-spot orgasm, there is a fifth kind of multiple:

5. **G-spot multiples:** Some women can only have multiple orgasms when they are receiving simultaneous clitoral and vaginal stimulation in the area of the G-spot.

What the Research Says

How Many Women Have Multiple Orgasms?

Theoretically, every woman can have multiple orgasms, because women, unlike men, do not have a refractory period following orgasm.

How many women actually do report having multiple orgasms?

Most surveys and studies cite that approximately 10 percent of women regularly experience multiples. Most of these women are in their thirties. Younger women have body or confidence issues that make orgasm more difficult for them. Women over forty might have less blood flow to the vagina, making repeated orgasm more difficult.

But women who began having multiple orgasms in their twenties are likely to keep having them into their forties and beyond.

How to Use the O Loop with Multiple Orgasm Techniques

The techniques for encouraging women's multiple orgasms were developed by Gina Ogden, Ph.D., therapist and author of the landmark book *Women Who Love Sex*, and the late Marc Meshorer, who, with his wife Judith, studied easily orgasmic women and contributed a great deal to our understanding of female sexuality.

The techniques are:

- Start on warm. Fantasize about the sexual encounter before it begins. Masturbate, but not to orgasm. You should be aroused to the point where the first orgasm will occur soon after lovemaking begins.
- Alternate stimuli. During lovemaking, alternate physical stimuli. The first one or two orgasms, for example, might be via cunnilingus or manual stimulation. Rarely will a woman have multiples if sex moves from foreplay straight to intercourse.

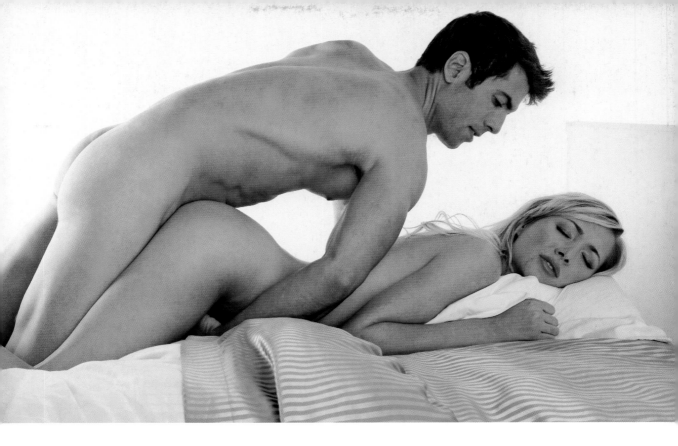

- Use your hands. Touch that clitoris! When you aren't stroking your clitoris, your lover probably should be. Don't leave your clitoris alone too long if you want to reach orgasm multiple times.
- Go for G-spot multiples. If you are G-spot responsive, have your partner use his fingers to stimulate your G-spot during cunnilingus; get into intercourse positions, especially rear entry, that favor G-spot stimulation; and add a G-spot vibrator to sex play.

HOW YOUR PARTNER CAN HELP

Here's how your partner can help stimulate G-spot multiples:

- He (or she) uses his (or her) fingers to stimulate the front wall of your vagina while performing cunnilingus, or

- He (or she) stimulates your clitoris during intercourse in a position that gives you G- spot stimulation.

The Secret to Multiples

All these techniques are good, and they are compatible with the Orgasm Loop.

Once you have mastered the O Loop, you can have multiple orgasms using it any time you want. The secret to multiples is keeping your arousal level high between orgasms. You can do that by sustaining your fire breathing and PC flexing through orgasm—and not stopping. If you do lose focus, go back to your arousal image and energy focus.

When you've just started O Looping, learning to reliably achieve one orgasm during sex may seem like enough of a goal for now. Don't write off the idea of multiples, though. After you have been using the Loop for a while, multiple orgasms will probably come more easily for you. And once you've experienced them, you may never be content with just one again.

TELL YOUR LOVER TO PRACTICE "THE FLAME"

For some women, this is the ultimate cunnilingus stroke.

Pretend the tip of your tongue is a candle flame. In your mind's eye, see that flame flickering in the wind. Move your tongue rapidly around the sides of her clitoris, above and below it, as the candle flame moves.

Real Talk

"I have had them on occasion. For me, the emotional element
has to be in place, too. I can come when I am not feeling
connected to my lover. But to have multiples, I need to feel close
to him. I can do that with the O Loop, but I don't have multiples
unless I feel that way."

—Tina, 33

"No. I am absolutely thrilled to have one now with the O Loop.
Maybe I will venture out into deeper waters soon."

—Vanessa, 23

"Yes. I learned how to have them while masturbating in my
twenties. The O Loop makes it even easier. I can come and
come until I just decide, 'Okay, I need to stop and do something
else now.'"

—Margo, 48

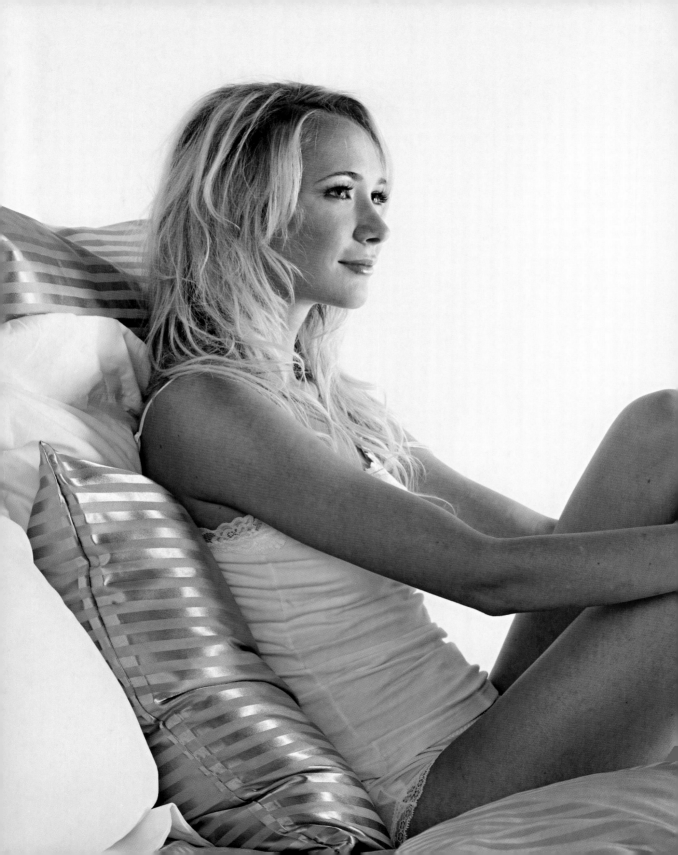

Part 5

The Special Needs O Loop

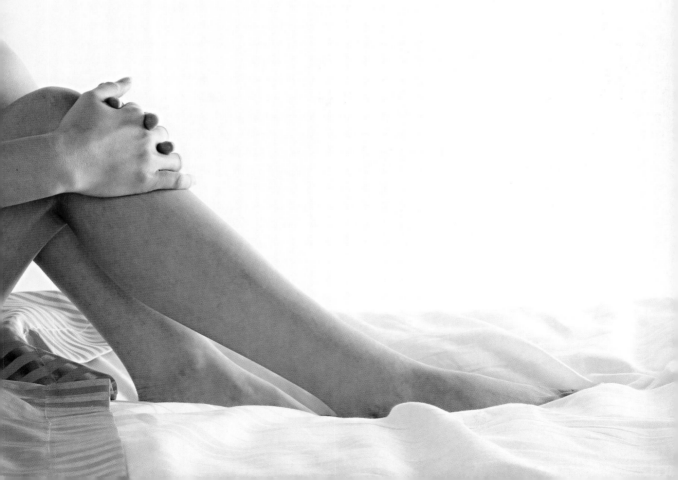

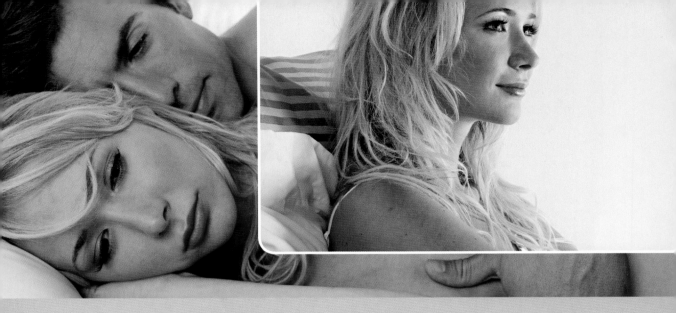

Chapter 6

The O Loop on Prozac

"SSRIs are wreaking havoc on human courtship. Women on these medications lose their ability to orgasm. Orgasm triggers the release of the hormone oxytocin—linked with pair bonding. So women who can't orgasm may be at a disadvantage in bonding and mating."

—Helen Fisher, Ph.D., anthropologist and author of *Why We Love: The Nature and Chemistry of Romantic Love*

MILLIONS OF WOMEN say they have low or no desire for sex and also experience difficulty reaching orgasm, if they can get there at all.

Millions of women take antidepressants daily.

There is a connection. Doctors and researchers acknowledge that the increase in low desire correlates with the introduction of a group of antidepressants called SSRIs (selective serotonin reuptake inhibitors) in the 1980s. Approximately 70 percent of men and women on SSRIs—and there are more women than men—suffer from sexual side effects. The women who take these medications often believe that low desire and orgasm difficulties are insurmountable obstacles to a good sex life.

And who can blame them for feeling that they must choose medication or orgasms? They've been given little support and encouragement from the medical establishment for overcoming the roadblocks to pleasure. But women should not have to choose between antidepressants and a good sex life. There are ways around this problem. Some antidepressants are less likely to have the side effect of loss of desire, and sometimes dosages can be changed to diminish that side effect. But the patient has to be assertive with her doctor in addressing the issue.

Some experts believe that antidepressants are overprescribed in Western countries, particularly the United States. That may be true. Undoubtedly, however, many people do benefit from taking Prozac, Zoloft, and other SSRI drugs. If you are one of them, you may think that your sex life has to be sacrificed for the greater good of your mental and emotional health. It doesn't.

The Orgasm Loop can help you become fully aroused and reach orgasm even if the medications you are taking have made that difficult.

Your Sexual Brain on Antidepressants

Antidepressants are not the only cause of low desire and orgasm difficulties. Chronic stress; poor body image; and medical issues, including pain, side effects of the birth control pill, and relationship problems, are among the other factors that negatively impact sexual response. But SSRIs are unique in the way they repress the chemicals of attraction and desire, dull some nerves associated with arousal, and inhibit orgasm.

They almost act as a buffer between you and your sexuality.

Talking to Your Doctor

Researchers have only recently begun to realize that the sexual side effects of antidepressants may not be the same for women and men. Many doctors don't ask patients about their sex lives. And patients too often are uncomfortable about bringing up the subject. Break the silence! Make an appointment with your doctor specifically to discuss the sexual side effects of your medication.

For some patients, switching antidepressants restores sexual function. For others, a lower dosage helps. In some cases, doctors prescribe "drug holidays"—physician-directed medication breaks—that allow patients to enjoy a sex break.

But do not stop medication on your own. It's never a good idea to stop medication abruptly without a doctor's guidance. Halting meds can also have side effects. With SSRIs in particular, medication dosages are (in most cases) gradually lowered.

What the Research Says

THE MISSING LOVE CONNECTION

Dopamine is one of the brain's natural feel-good chemicals. According to Dr. Helen Fisher and her research partner psychiatrist Andrew Thomson, when SSRIs suppress dopamine, it affects sexual response in several ways. By suppressing dopamine, drugs like Prozac block a person's ability to have the feelings of elation and ecstasy that accompany falling in love. They might not feel the spark that should ignite when they meet a person who is a good match for them. If they do have a partner, low desire and orgasm difficulties can take a toll on the relationship.

"SSRIs interrupt the flow of chemicals that help us fall and stay in love," Fisher says. Most of us don't realize how dependent "love" is on brain chemicals. Having sex when you are chemically impaired is like eating when you have a bad head cold: Something is missing.

SEXERCISES TO STIMULATE THE PELVIC REGION

If you are having arousal issues, these two sexercises will help stimulate
the sexual nerve endings in your pelvic region.

The Sexy Squat

Stand with your feet shoulder-width apart and slowly lower your butt as if
you were going to sit in a chair. Squeeze your PC muscle and the muscles in
your buttocks as you rise back up. Do three times daily.

The Seat

Sit back on your heels and reach your arms forward. Hold for one minute,
then sit up and lean back as far as you can, hands on the floor behind you
for support. Hold for one minute. Do three times daily.

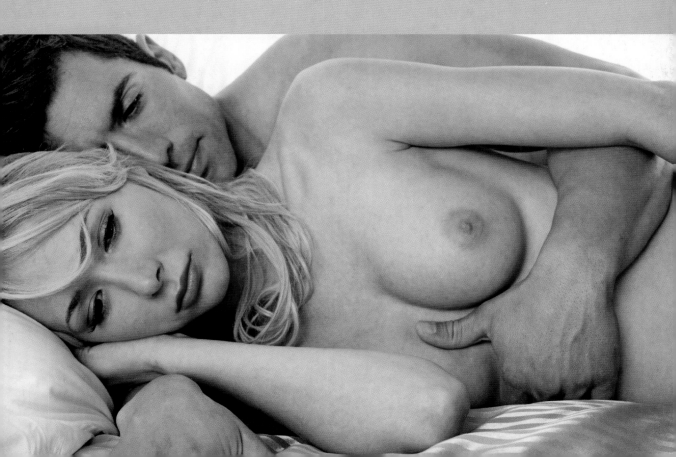

Real Talk

"I went on Zoloft for postpartum depression and stayed on it for over a year. I had no sex drive. When I would have sex to please my husband, I rarely got aroused. And I did not have an orgasm the whole time. It almost wrecked our marriage."

—Lana, 31

"I've been on antidepressants off and on for several years. They did kill my libido. I could reach orgasm on the rare occasions I had sex—if I had an understanding partner willing to put in the time. My doctor switched me to Wellbutrin, which has fewer sexual side effects. Now I am in a relationship and using the O Loop to get aroused and reach orgasm.

—Noelle, 39

"My doctor put me on antidepressants after I lost my husband to a younger woman, my job to a corporate takeover, and my mother to cancer—all in one year. I took the pills for eight months before I realized that they were taking something else from me—my sexuality. In my case, antidepressants weren't necessary. I needed a good cry, and they even kept me from having that. Participating in the O Loop study was my first step back to feeling good."

—Janice, 51

How the O Loop Can Lessen the Impact of Antidepressants

The O Loop will work for you the same way it does for women who aren't on SSRIs—it will just take longer. Your sexual nerve pathways may be dulled, but they aren't dead. Research has shown that women with spinal cord injuries experience orgasm in the brain when they are mentally and emotionally aroused and receiving stimulation to any part of the body. Women can reach orgasm via four pathways to the brain, including the vagus nerve, which connects the vagina directly to the brain, thus bypassing the spinal cord. The power of the mind is great, and we are only beginning to realize how great. And the O Loop begins in your head.

Here's how to make the O Loop work for you:

1. **Use a vibe first.**

   Choose an external vibe. Use it on your genitals for several minutes until you feel sexually stimulated. Turn it off.

2. **Meditate on your arousal image.**

   Get into your arousal image as described in Chapter 2.

3. **Focus your sexual energy.**

   Follow the directions in Chapter 2. Don't be discouraged if you don't feel that energy quickly. Keep focusing until you do.

4. **Turn on the vibe again.**

   Add the fire breathing and PC flexing techniques described in Chapter 2. When you have established a good rhythm, pick up the vibe.

5. **Don't worry about orgasm now.**

   It will happen. You may not come the first or second time you use the O Loop. If you're tired, quit—but not in frustration. Enjoy the sensations you are feeling. Your body is aroused; you are responding sexually. And the orgasm will happen.

"JUST DO IT" is one of the best pieces of sex advice you'll ever get, whether you are on medications or not. Don't say no to sex with your partner because you're "not in the mood." Do it anyway. Use the O Loop and concentrate on becoming aroused, staying aroused, and feeling your sexual power return. Don't worry about reaching orgasm. Having more frequent sex—with or without orgasm—will cause those suppressed chemicals of desire to start flowing again. THAT IS TRUE FOR ALL OF US.

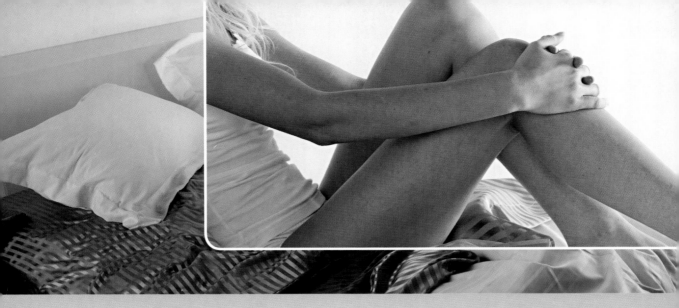

Chapter 7

The Aging O Loop—After 40 and More

"Sex is more honest at midlife. There are so many things you can say and do that you couldn't say and do before."

—Lionel Shriver, author of *The Post-Birthday World* and other novels

IN THEIR TWENTIES, women are the most coveted objects of desire for men of all ages. In their thirties, they reach orgasm more easily and more often. In their forties, they have greater confidence in their sexual abilities and luxuriate in their power. If you think it is all over for women at fifty or even sixty, you must be very young. With cover babes like Goldie Hawn, Michelle Pfeiffer, Sharon Stone, and others, the aging baby boom generation has changed the sexual status quo that valued older men and wrote off older women as "dried up." Women of all ages now will benefit from this new perspective on female sexual evolution

Changes that impact negatively on sexuality do occur in the body at midlife. Emotional and psychological issues, such as fear of aging and unhappiness with a partner, also take their toll on desire and arousal. But remedies exist for all these problems, and there are midlife blessings and benefits, other positive physical, mental, and emotional changes that make sex a more rewarding experience. And using the Orgasm Loop during masturbation and lovemaking can give you some of the best orgasms of your life.

Midlife Sex Issues

Physical and psychological changes at midlife do impact our sex lives. Both men and women, for example, need more physical stimulation to become aroused. Some of the changes, especially in women, are beneficial ones.

Your Sex Drive Isn't What It Used to Be

Estrogen and testosterone levels and the adrenal gland hormone DHEA all decline as we age, and those declining hormone levels are usually blamed for a low libido. Other factors that can also contribute to a drop in sex drive include a sedentary lifestyle, weight gain, health problems, and relationship issues. And that last one is significant. Couples who have been in a monogamous relationship for years often have unresolved conflicts and repressed anger. A woman may be disappointed in her husband's lovemaking, especially if the rut they are in doesn't include regular orgasms for her.

Your Genitals (or Your Partner's) Aren't Responsive

In midlife, women experience reduced blood flow to the clitoris and vagina. That, accompanied by declining hormone levels, has a negative impact on the vagina. Women complain about insufficient lubrication. They may not realize their vaginas have also lost some elasticity and that they have some decrease in genital sensitivity. The two big factors—dryness and inelasticity—can make intercourse uncomfortable. If the dryness and inelasticity are severe, intercourse is painful and can cause bleeding.

Suffering their own testosterone loss and reduced blood flow to the genitals, male partners may have difficulty getting and sustaining a solid erection.

You Have Body Anxiety

It's hard to age gracefully in a society where thirty-year-old women are getting Botox injections at the first sign of a wrinkle and midlife role models are surgically enhanced.

Some women in midlife do feel the pressure of unrealistic expectations on aging. But, ironically, the weight of unrealistic expectations falls hardest on younger women today. Their aging mothers and older sisters are benefiting from the positive new slant the media has put on aging women. But younger women are left to struggle with the ever increasing pressure of unrealistic beauty and youth standards that are presently being imposed on women at a younger and younger age.

You Have Health Problems

Chronic pain, medical conditions like high blood pressure and diabetes, fibroids, and other conditions can seem like sex-life terminators, especially if you don't have a man who has made that "in sickness and in health" pledge. Medications (especially antidepressants, as discussed in the previous chapter) can affect sexual function, too.

You Have Money Concerns

Studies have shown that sexual dysfunction is highest in women with poor health and/or money problems. (And if you have poor health, you probably have a money problem, too.) Midlife divorce, corporate downsizing, and the cost of educating children put many women in this age group into a compromised financial situation.

What the Research Says

SEXUAL SIDE EFFECTS

Don't count on your doctor to tell you about the sexual side effects of medications or the impact of disease on your sexuality.

A 2007 survey conducted by The Women's Sexual Health Foundation found that less than 8 percent of women are asked about their sex lives by their health care providers during annual visits. Yet 80 percent of women believe that their OB-GYNs have the knowledge and training to help them with sexual problems.

You have to bring up the subject of your sex life. Being responsible for your own orgasms extends beyond the bedroom and into the consultation room. When talking with your doctors, don't be embarrassed to be assertive about the importance of sex in your life.

The Usually Prescribed Fixes

Some of the treatments for midlife sex issues do help. They include:

- Hormone Replacement Therapy (HRT) for women, and testosterone replacement for men. (Caveat: Be aware that for several years there has been and continues to be controversy over the safety and desirability of using HRT. Before beginning such treatments, be sure to do as much research on your own as possible and then discuss your options thoroughly with your doctor.)
- Lubricants, including some long-lasting lubricants. Replens and KY Liquid Beads are two good products that last for two or three days if used regularly.
- Kegels and Kegel exercisers (see Chapter 2 for more information).
- More healthful diets and exercise programs.
- Adjustments to lovemaking styles that include more, and more varied, genital stroking, alterations to intercourse positions, more oral sex, and more frequent sex.
- Vibrators.
- Herbal treatments (but do your research on these products, because they are not regulated by the FDA and many make false claims).

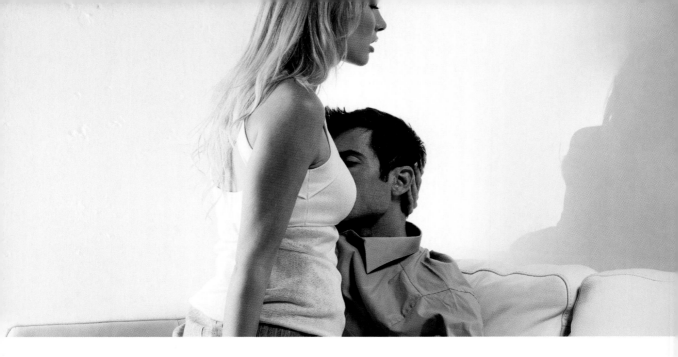

How the O Loop Can Help You Overcome Midlife Sex Issues

You may not be distracted by babies and small children anymore, but you, like younger women, have a lot on your mind besides sex. Often, you need help in focusing your arousal, too. Even though orgasm is more reliable in midlife women who have regular sex, it's not a sure thing if you can't sustain arousal.

The Orgasm Loop works because it:

- Stimulates arousal (by using an arousal image).
- Increases blood flow to the genitals through energy focus and fire breathing.
- Improves genital and pelvic conditioning through PC flexing.
- Makes orgasm more likely and orgasms stronger.

Use the O Loop during masturbation (including with a vibrator) and during lovemaking. After you've been using it for a few weeks, you will feel like your younger sexual self—only better. At midlife, women have greater self-confidence, less fear about sex and intimacy, less need to "please" all the time, and more willingness to try something new.

With the help of the Orgasm Loop, you can have it all—a more youthful sexual response and the sassy attitude to go with it.

Real Talk

HOW IS YOUR SEX LIFE?

"Much better than I expected it to be at this point in my life! I've been married to the same man for forty years. Our passion has waxed and waned over the years. Our bodies have shifted. But we do have an active and satisfying sex life. We stay in shape and try to be open to new ideas—like the O Loop, which has increased my clitoral sensitivity and made my orgasms stronger."

—Barbara, 60

"My sex life is great. I am in a new marriage after being divorced for three years. I read somewhere that the age of the relationship affects sex more than the age of the lovers—and that's been true with us. We can't get enough of each other. The O Loop put the icing on my cake. I have learned how to have multiple orgasms."

—Nicola, 51

"I have had some orgasm issues most of my life. I've always been able to orgasm—and many times—while masturbating, but couldn't put it together with most of my lovers. It really only worked for me if they had gifted tongues. Using the O Loop, I've been able to come during intercourse. It's thrilling."

—Pam, 54

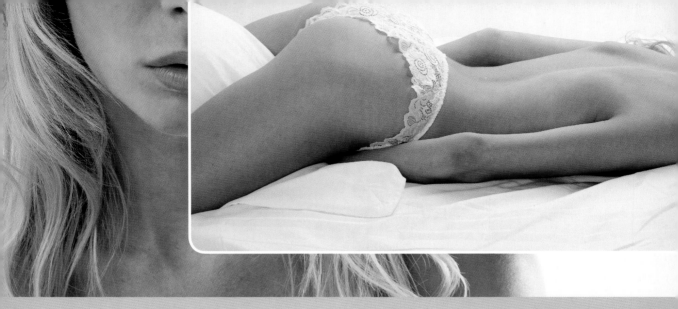

Chapter 8
The Celibate O Loop

"Don't knock masturbation. It's sex with someone I love."

—Woody Allen (as the character Alvey Singer) in the movie *Annie Hall*

EVEN THOUGH WOMEN are the gender who can always get laid, most of us will experience a sexual partner drought—and likely more than one—at some point in our lives. There are many reasons why women might find themselves on their own at certain points in their lives, including these:

- Our hearts are wounded. We're just out of one relationship and are not ready for another.
- We're too picky. None of the men (women) we meet appeal to us right now.
- They're too picky. No one we want wants us.
- We have no time! We are working twelve hours a day, or raising a child alone, or finishing our medical residency.
- We are healing—from an STD, cancer treatment, the death of our mother.

And there are, of course, even more reasons than these.

A time alone need not, and should not, be a time without sex. Sexuality is part of our vitality, our life force. We can't shut that down without suffering the repercussions, such as jumping into bed with a totally inappropriate man because we're desperate or, post-menopause, feeling our vaginas wither.

While you're between lovers, love yourself.

The Orgasm Loop can help you nurture, even expand, that self-love, which in turn will make you more loving and lovable when the drought ends.

Why You Need to Stay Sexually Active When You're Alone

Step 1 of the O Loop technique makes the case for the physical benefits of masturbation, whether you have a partner or not. Yes, masturbation is good for your body. And it's good for your sexual mind.

If you're going through a celibate phase, you need to masturbate for all those benefits, and more. Use this time and the Orgasm Loop to expand your sexuality so that you will be more responsive, orgasmic, creative, and erotically adventurous when you take the next lover into your bed.

You can expand your sexuality by:

- Fantasizing.
- Extending the time that orgasm lasts.
- Spreading orgasm throughout your whole body.
- Expanding orgasm beyond the genitals.
- Playing with new sex toys that stimulate you in different ways.

Why Fantasize?

Fantasy is a nearly universal experience, a mental aphrodisiac that is sometimes a conscious process, sometimes not. Recent studies indicate that men and women now have fantasies that are more alike than they were twenty years ago. According to Nancy Friday, author of *Women on Top* and other books about sexual fantasies, women's fantasies have become more graphic and overtly sexual and aggressive. Don't be afraid or ashamed of these fantasies. Use them and don't take them too seriously. When you're alone, your fantasies will likely be richer because you won't be thinking about a man, or feeling guilty because you're not thinking about him.

What Is an Extended Orgasm?

The average orgasm has three to five contractions and maybe some aftershocks. An extended orgasm may have anywhere from five to twenty contractions, with the last few feeling slower and drawn out, but definitely not aftershocks. Extended orgasms are more likely to occur when you have time for slow, languorous masturbation (or lovemaking), the kind of sex that keeps you feeling "on the verge" for a long time before orgasm begins.

To try it, masturbate in a comfortable position using the Orgasm Loop. Keep the PC flexing and fire breathing going continuously through orgasm rather than stopping when you feel the first contraction. Your orgasm will extend (and may turn into extended multiple orgasms).

Real Talk

"If I don't have a partner, I don't think about sex very often.
Maybe I don't let myself think about it. When I feel horny,
I masturbate. Pretty soon, somebody appealing comes along."

—Molly, 34

"Call an old sex buddy. It's better than nothing."

—Tiffany, 26

"Masturbate, masturbate, masturbate! I don't masturbate when
I'm in a relationship. And I'm damned good, too. I cheat myself
out of a lot of good sex when I'm with a man."

—Carla, 42

"I indulge my sensual side. Bubble baths, champagne for one,
vibrator time."

—Chloe, 33

The Whole-Body Orgasm

Occasionally, an orgasm is both intense and diffuse. The tremors seem to radiate out from the genitals to the far reaches of the body's extremities. You feel it blowing out the top of your head and out through your toes.

Some people experience whole-body orgasms only when they have a strong emotional connection to their partners. For others, it occurs when they are feeling particularly sensual or sexual or both. Use this time alone to find your way more deeply into your sexual self and into the whole-body orgasm.

To try it, masturbate in a comfortable position using the O Loop. As soon as your energy is concentrated in your genitals, use your hand to massage your vulva, inner thighs, and groin with light, shallow strokes in time with fire breathing and PC flexing. Imagine that you are spreading arousal throughout those areas. Continue the massage during your orgasm, imagining that you are spreading the orgasm throughout your body.

Extragenital Orgasm

An extragenital orgasm is triggered by stimulation to any part of the body except the genitals. If you have experienced multiple and/or extended orgasms, you will be able to come this way, too. Women who have mastered the O Loop are more likely to have this kind of orgasm because energy focus, fire breathing, and PC flexing stimulate the genitals without direct physical contact.

A woman who is proficient at using the O Loop can have a no-hands orgasm any way. So why wouldn't she be able to orgasm from breast play?

Playing with Toys

I am enthusiastic about sex toys for every woman, but especially women alone. In general, women are too serious about sex, making it all about love and relationship and commitment. When you're alone with your toys it's all about the play, the sex. Here are some suggestions:

1. **Make dildos your friend.**

    Why bother when they don't vibrate? You can control the speed and motion of the thrusting with your hand. And using a dildo may seem more like intercourse, especially if you select a dildo made of lifelike materials and in sizes that penises actually come in. Huge dildos are more for show than insertion. (If you want to play with one, use it to stroke your vulva, labia, and clitoris.)

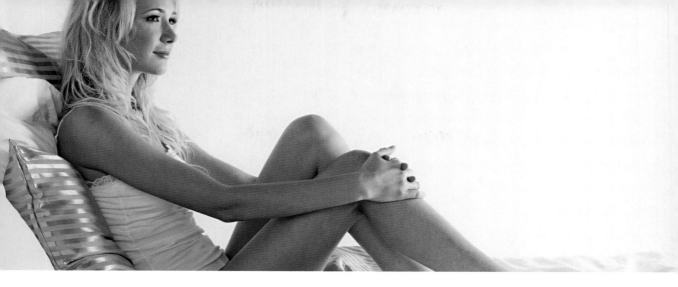

"After my divorce, I had the best sex I'd had in years—with myself. I bought seven vibrators, one for every night of the week. And I watched the kind of porn that I like."

—Deborah, 46

2. **Erotic DVDs and videos are sex toys, too.** They are often used to stimulate arousal during masturbation. And many couples use them as part of foreplay or to improve technique and learn new ways of having sex. Masturbate with the O Loop while watching a film. Match your fire breathing and PC flexing rhythm to the action.

3. **Anal toys are worth experimenting with, too.** Sex toys are a good way to prepare for anal intercourse. Or you can use them for anal masturbation. They include:

    Butt plugs: Also called anal plugs, they are typically diamond-shaped with a thin neck and a flared base, which prevents them from slipping into the rectum.

O LOOP FANTASIZING

Here are some tips to get your creative energy flowing anytime:

- Let your mind drift into a fantasy, perhaps inspired by a book or film.

- When you feel slightly aroused, shift to your arousal image as if you were flipping channels on the television.

- Once you are fully aroused and your energy is focused, return to that fantasy.

- Adjust the rhythm of your fire breathing and PC flexing to the sexual activity in your fantasy.

What the Research Says

ORGASM WITHOUT GENITAL STIMULATION

Between 1 and 3 percent of women—and almost no men—can reach orgasm without genital stimulation. When it does occur, extragenital orgasm usually follows one orgasm (or more) triggered the old-fashioned way, via the genitals. A highly orgasmic woman, for example, can reach the third, fourth, or fifth orgasm by having her breasts or nipples stroked, sucked, pinched, pulled, or massaged. Some women at that point can even come by squeezing their thighs together.